Care of the Older Person

Edited by
Rob Garbett, RGN, BN

Illustrated by
Peter Gardiner

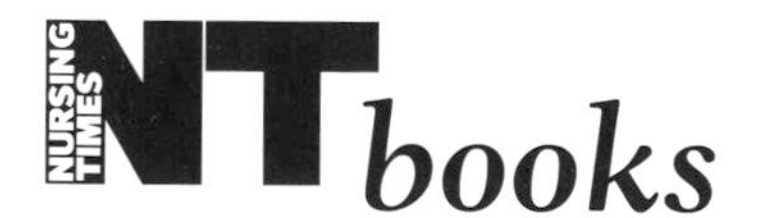

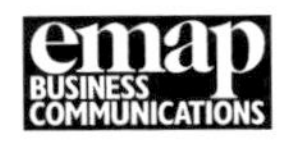

Published by
Emap Healthcare, part of Emap Business Communications Ltd
Greater London Road,
Hampstead Road
London NW1 7EJ

Companies and representatives throughout the world
Film output (repro) by Prepress Services, Leeds, West Yorkshire
Printed in Great Britain by Drogher Press, Christchurch, Dorset

ISBN 1 902499 19 0

Contents

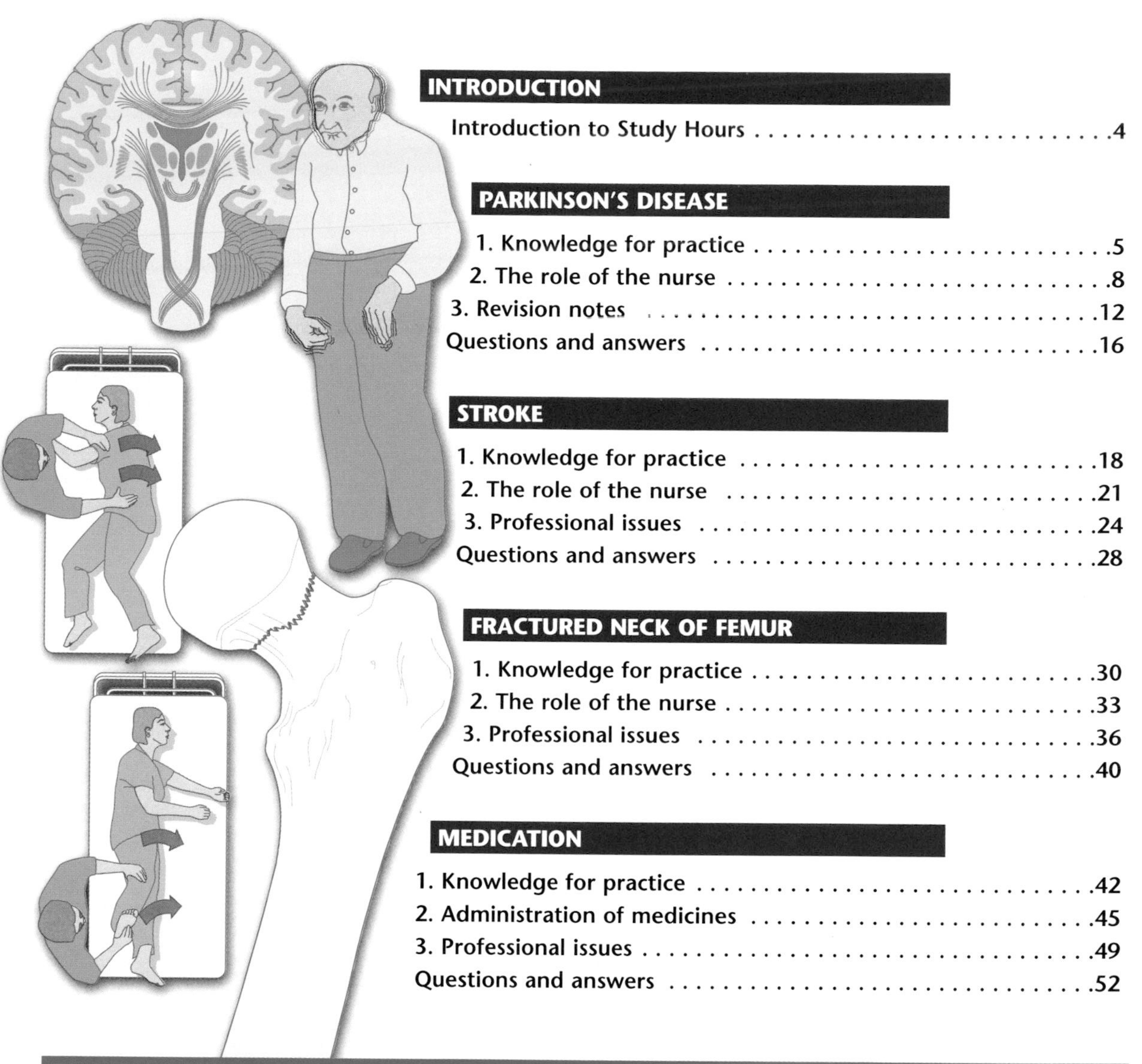

CONTRIBUTORS

Parkinson's disease:
Author: Nevin Stewart, RGN, DipN, nurse development manager, Moseley Hospital NHS Trust, Surrey

Stroke:
Authors: Brian Booth, RGN, MRSH, projects manager, *Nursing Times* Projects Team; Ann Warren, RGN, ward manager, Redwood Stroke Unit, Tolworth Hospital, Surbiton

Fractured neck of femur:
Authors: Melanie Fisher, BSc(Hons), RGN, ONC, DPSN, practice development nurse, surgical directorate, The Royal Victoria Infirmary NHS Trust, Newcastle-upon-Tyne; Mark Mowatt, RN, DipHE, staff nurse, orthopaedic/trauma department, Newcastle General Hospital; Adam Legge

Medication:
Author: Martin Shepherd, BPharm, MSc, MRPharmS, head of Pharmacy Services, Chesterfield and North Derbyshire Royal Hospital NHS Trust, Chesterfield

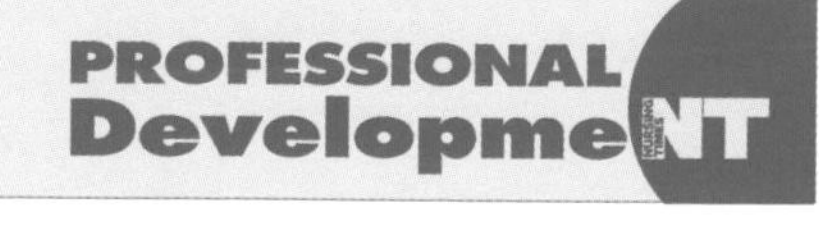

Keep yourself up to date

Use your reading as a vital part of your professional updating

Welcome to *Nursing Times'* Professional Development Book 4. It follows on from our popular Professional Development *Nursing Times* series (PDNT), which ran for over three years.

The contents have been revised and updated to ensure that they reflect contemporary thinking in the areas concerned. The books are designed for busy clinical nurses looking to update their knowledge and skills, for students and for practitioners returning to work after a break.

Each unit concludes with a multiple choice questionnaire for you to test your knowledge. This book and others in the series provide you with one means to keep up to date and relate your learning practice so that you can meet the UKCC's standards for post registration education (PREP).

This book uses *Nursing Times* Study Hours help you keep a record of what you learn and how long it took you.

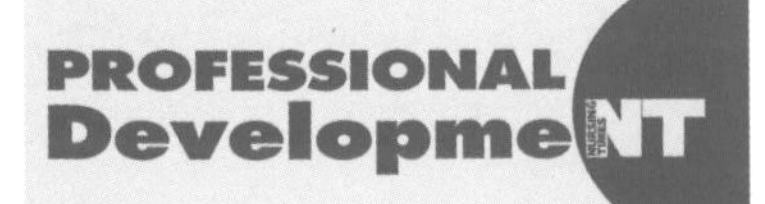

PREP MADE SIMPLE

STUDY HOURS

Lifelong learning is an important part of every nurse's working life. The UKCC has provided a framework to help nurses relate their learning to practice in order to provide safe and effective practice.

While there has been a degree of anxiety about how to meet the minimum requirement of five days study or its equivalent, we at *Nursing Times* believe that reading the professional press can be of great help.

Study Hours have been designed by *Nursing Times* to provide an easy-to-use estimation of the time you spend reflecting on and studying clinical issues. Using Study Hours puts you in control of your own professional development and helps you meet the PREP requirements.

THE STUDY HOURS RATING

The Study Hours rating is the figure inside the clock. It is our estimate of the number of hours it will take you to read and reflect on the material provided.

The figure given is our estimate but it does not matter if you take more or less time; record the time you spend in your professional profile.

STUDY 3 HOURS

STUDY HOURS IN PRACTICE

Reading articles, supplements and publications such as this can be a passive affair but it can also, if you choose, be the starting point of a great deal of reflection and practice-related activity.

For example, imagine a nurse in a genito-urinary clinic reading something in *NT* about dying with dignity: an article looking at different cultural beliefs surrounding death. Although working with death is not usually a feature of her working day, the nurse realises that sexuality and sexual taboos are very significant in the location where she works, which has a large population from an Asian background. The nurse realises that despite this, relatively few Asian clients present at her clinic so she investigates further to find out what social and cultural factors might be at work. As a result of her research the nurse is able to establish an outreach network with local community centres, social clubs and places of work where she gives talks and hands out information in a number of languages stressing the need for early investigation and treatment of genito-urinary disease.

All this activity represents activity relevant to meeting PREP requirements and comes from reading the professional press. We hope that the materials in the book will similarly stimulate your personal and professional development.

The Study Hours logo is a registered trade mark of Emap Healthcare Ltd

Parkinson's disease

Knowledge for practice

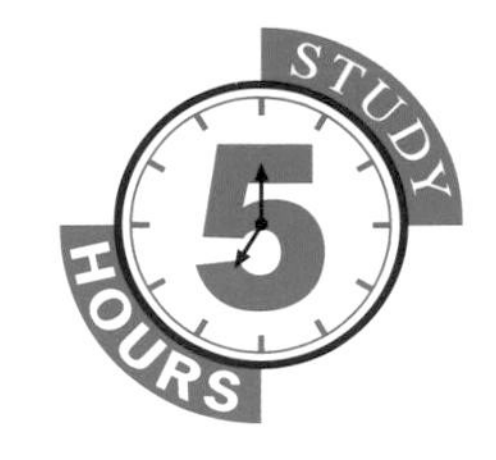

Parkinson's disease (PD) has potentially profound effects on every aspect of daily living in those diagnosed with the disorder.

KEY FEATURES OF PARKINSON'S DISEASE

PD is a disorder of movement and posture first recognised by James Parkinson in 1817 and reported in his paper *Essay on the Shaking Palsy*. Parkinson described six patients in whom there was a combination of 'involuntary tremulous movement' and a characteristic gait disorder.

Other features have subsequently been added to this original description; thus, the diagnosis of PD is based on the existence of a combination of these clinical features (Sagar, 1991; MacMahon, 1990).

Normally there is a balance between the chemical messengers acetycholine (excitatory) and dopamine (inhibitory) in the nervous system. In PD a lack of dopamine causes slowness, an overbalance of acetycholine causes tremor and the imbalance between the two causes stiffness. Death of dopamine cells happens more rapidly in PD than people without the disease, patients with parkinsonian symptoms presenting when approximately 80% of dopamine loss has occurred (Roberts et al, 1993). What causes this is unknown but a wide variety of agents have been considered, from infectious, toxic and other exposures. It is now known that non-smokers have a greater risk of disease although the reason for this is unclear (Birtwistle and Hall, 1996). People exposed to pesticides and with head injury also show a consistently elevated risk but are prone to biased measurement. Hereditary factors, although originally discounted, have recently emerged as a focus of PD research (Polymeropoulos, 1998). It is likely that the cause is multifactorial, with contributions of variable significance from genetic predisposition, environmental toxins and ageing.

Parkinsonism and PD are found throughout the world. Prevalence increases with age without significant differences between the sexes. Mortality and incidence data suggest that the disease may be less common today in younger age groups, symptoms usually occurring after the age of 50 (Ben-Shlomo, 1997). In the UK the most recent estimates of overall prevalence of PD have been 140–160 per 100,000 population — a GP's list of 2,000 will have about three PD patients. Along with stroke and osteoarthritis, it is one of the most frequently physically disabling conditions of older people. However, a substantial proportion of patients with PD go undetected in the general population.

The underlying pathological abnormality is a loss of pigmentation in the substantia nigra of the basal ganglia of the brain (Fig 1). This is related to a depletion in the neurotransmitter dopamine in this area. The basal ganglia form part of the extrapyramidal system, which controls movement and posture, and the depletion in dopamine

Fig 1. Cross-section of the brain showing areas involved in Parkinson's disease

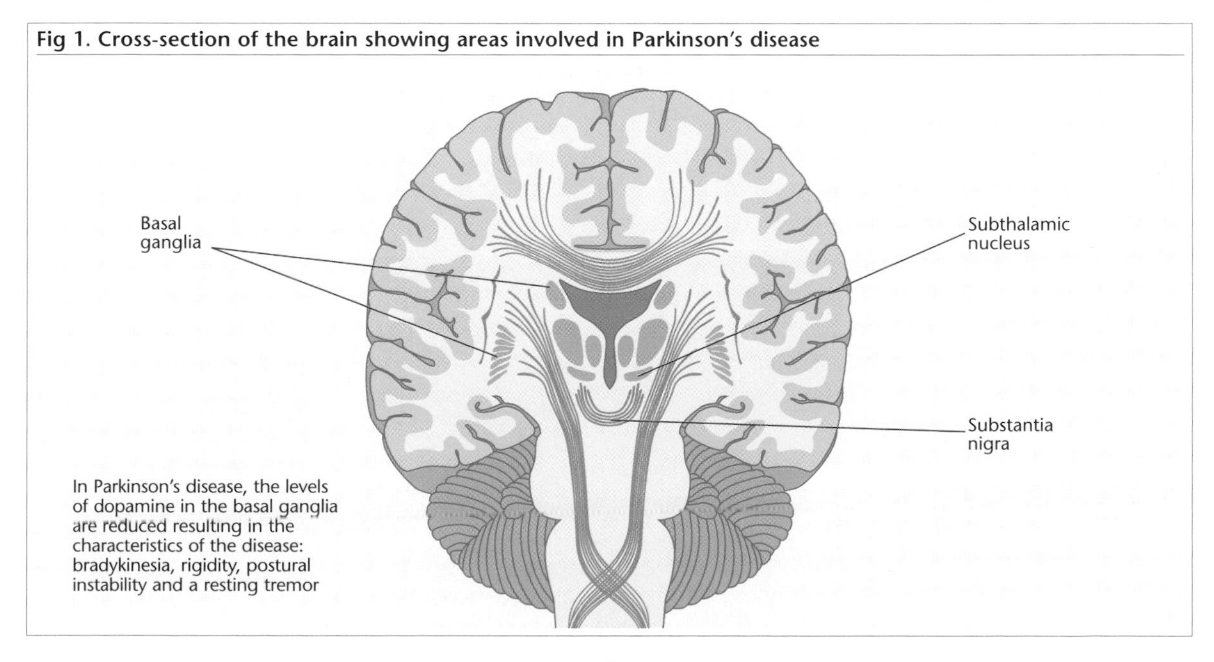

BTable 1. Key clinical features of Parkinson's disease

The appearance of patients with Parkinson's disease can be explained by the presence of two or more of the following clinical features:

- Bradykinesia
- Muscular rigidity
- Resting tremor
- Postural instability

Glossary

Akinesia
Complete lack of movement: an extreme form of bradykinesia

Antimuscarinic or anticholinergic drugs
Drugs such as benzhexol used in the treatment of Parkinson's disease. They work by blocking the action of the neurotransmitter acetylcholine

Apraxia
Loss of ability to carry out skilled movements

Basal ganglia
Part of the nervous system that coordinates movement — the main damaged area in Parkinson's disease

Bradykinesia
Slow initiation of voluntary movements

Dyskinesia
Twitching, fidgeting, withering or flapping (involuntary) movements that occur usually as a side-effect of levadopa treatment

Dystonia
An involuntary sustained contraction of one set of muscles; similar to spasm

Festinating gait
The typical gait of Parkinson's disease in which the person makes a series of rapid short steps

Freezing
A sudden unpredictable akinesia that usually occurs during walking

Methyl-phenyl-tetrahydropyridine (MPTP)
A poisonous substance that damages the nerve cells of the substantia nigra and produces a condition virtually indistinguishable from Parkinson's disease

Rigidity
Stiffness of the muscles: one of the main signs of Parkinson's disease

Substantia nigra
Part of the basal ganglia involved in coordinating movement

Tremor
Involuntary shaking of the limbs and head; tremor is common but does not occur in every patient

results in slowing of movement (bradykinesia). Drug therapy for PD attempts to replace the effect of dopamine in the substantia nigra.

PARKINSONISM

Several other conditions can mimic PD but the underlying pathological processes are different. Parkinsonism is a term used to describe the symptoms of PD, which can be divided into four categories:

- Primary or idiopathic: PD
- Secondary: drug-induced (due to neuroleptics, some antiemetics, MPTP) trauma, stroke, tumour
- Parkinson's-plus syndromes, for example multiple system atrophy, progressive supranuclear palsy, Shy Drager syndrome, Lewy body disease
- Hereditary degenerative disease, for example, Huntington's disease, Wilson's disease

KEY CLINICAL FEATURES (TABLE 1)

Bradykinesia

Bradykinesia is a slowness of movement with difficulty in initiating activities. Patients may also experience problems with, for example, getting up from a chair and turning over in bed at night (with subsequent risk of pressure sores in advanced disease).

Rigidity

Rigidity refers to increased tone in the muscles and leads to a stooped posture with legs and arms slightly flexed.

Tremor

The tremor in PD is characteristic but does not have to be present to make the diagnosis. The presence of tremor for other reasons is common (especially in older people) and can lead to errors in diagnosis.

In PD, tremor is present at rest and typically involves a 'pill-rolling' motion of the forefinger on the thumb. It is made worse by anxiety and tends to improve on voluntary movement. It may occur on one or both sides. Tremor may also be present in the head and neck.

Other tremors that may be confused with PD are those of cerebellar disease and essential tremor. Neither of these tends to be present at rest and both may be made worse with movement.

Postural instability

The difficulties experienced with control of fine movement result in problems with balance and control in movement. In turn this can increase the risk of falls (Quinn, 1995).

ONSET OF PARKINSON'S DISEASE

Initial onset of PD is gradual and symptoms may be present for a year or two before the diagnosis becomes clear. A coarse, one-sided resting tremor is a common neurological presentation but loss of use and reduced coordination

Fig 2. The clinical signs of Parkinson's disease

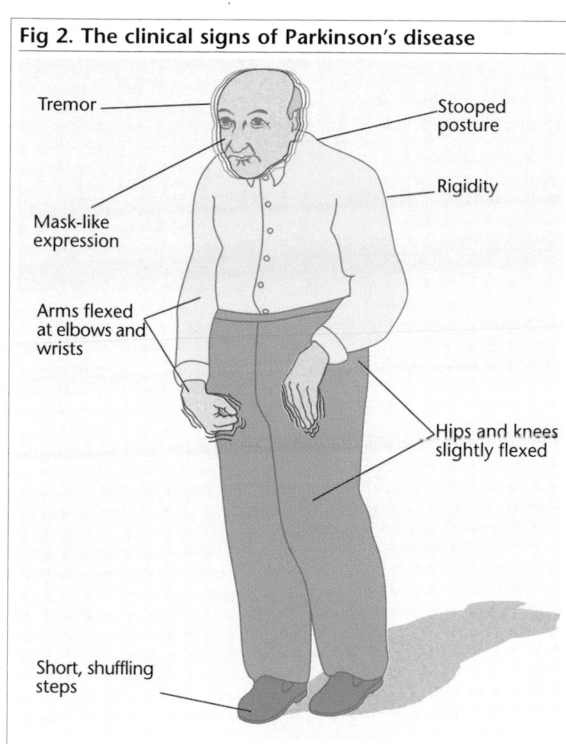

Table 2. Adverse effects of anti-parkinsonian drugs

L-dopa preparations
Nausea
Postural hypotension
Dyskinesia
Nightmares
Psychosis

Dopamine agonists
Nausea
Postural hypotension
Dyskinesia
Nightmares
Psychosis

Selegiline
Increases likelihood of adverse side-effects caused by L-dopa or dopamine agonists

Anticholinergic (antimuscarinic) drugs
Dry mouth (which can be beneficial where excess saliva production is a problem)
Constipation
Urinary retention
Confusion

down one side of the body may also occur and be mistaken for a hemiplegia. A dull ache in one shoulder or arm may occur, as may backache or pains in the legs. Depression may precede the disorder but symptoms of fatigue, loss of initiative and general slowing down are more common. Some patients may present with falls caused by loss of postural stability.

Once the disease is fully established there is a characteristic posture and gait and patients have more difficulty with initiating movement than maintaining it (Fig 2). They often find it difficult to start walking, but when they do walk it is with a hurrying (or festinating) gait, characterised by small steps leaning forward on the front part of the foot with the knees slightly bent. Because the heel rarely touches the floor, they may have difficulty stopping and risk falling. If stopped, patients may find it difficult to start again. There is also a loss of the normal involuntary swing of the arms on walking.

A person who has the disease may also present with infrequent blinking of the eyes and a loss of function in the facial muscles resulting in a 'mask-like' expression. The limbs may be affected by 'cogwheel' rigidity (rhythmic muscular contractions on passive movement) (MacMahon, 1995).

Diagnosis is made on the basis of the presence of bradykinesia plus at least one of the other key features. It may also be supported by the presence of some of the following less frequently encountered features:

- Seborrhoeic dermatitis: a condition causing greasy skin
- Dysphagia: difficulty with swallowing, which can cause chest infection subsequent to inhalation of food or fluid
- Constipation
- Excessive salivation, which, in combination with dysphagia, results in drooling of saliva
- Micrographia: a progressive reduction in the size of handwriting
- Anxiety
- Depression
- Mild or moderate dementia with the progression of the disease
- Dysphonia: reduction in volume of the voice with loss of variation in expression
- Postural hypotension: a fall in blood pressure when the patient stands up.

DRUG TREATMENT

Drug treatment for PD is aimed at compensating for the deficiency of dopamine in the brain. Dopamine cannot be given directly in its pure form as it does not pass from the bloodstream into the brain. It is therefore given as levadopa (L-Dopa), a compound which will pass into the brain where it is converted into dopamine.

The main types of drugs used to treat PD are:

- Levadopa (L-dopa), co-careldopa (Sinemet) and co-beneldopa (Madopar) are drugs that replace dopamine. They are given in combination with peripheral dopa-decarboxylase inhibitor in order for them to cross the blood-brain barrier and to help control some of the side-effects. This approach remains the single most effective one for the control of parkinsonism

- Dopamine agonists (that is, drugs which increase levels of dopamine); for example, bromocriptine, pergolide, lysuride and apomorphine
- The MAO-B (monoamine oxidase type B inhibitor), selegiline, prevents the breakdown of dopamine and can be used as monotherapy
- Anticholinergics, such as benzhexol, orphenadrine, procyclidine and benztrophine, dampen down the effects of acetycholine, helping to restore a balance with dopamine, improving tremor. Their usefulness is limited by side-effects, especially in older people, including confusion, dry mouth, blurred vision retention of urine and constipation.

Levadopa preparations

Most patients with PD, except perhaps those with very early or mild symptoms, will be taking an L-dopa preparation. It improves symptoms related to bradykinesia and rigidity but is less effective for controlling tremor.

Early side-effects of treatment include postural hypotension, sweating attacks, aggravation of peptic ulcers and confusion, but it is usually the long-term side-effects (manifesting after five to 10 years taking the drug) that are the most problematic.

RECENT ADVANCES

Dopamine agonists

These are apomorphine injection, bromocriptine, lisuride, pergolide, ropinirole, cabergoline and pramipexol, which first appeared in the early 1970s. They are compounds that mimic dopamine.

They are more receptor-site specific and have a longer half-life. Because of this the adverse effects of levodopa are minimised. Their exact role in the treatment of PD is controversial.

Much time is given to discussion as to their efficacy as adjunct therapy, monotherapy or neuroprotective therapy.

Catechol-O-methyltransferase (COMT) inhibitors

These agents inhibit the degradation of levodopa through the enzyme COMT. They were launched in 1998. Tolcapone was withdrawn in late 1998 and entacapone is now the only one available on the UK market.

Drug regimens

The decision to initiate treatment is somewhat controversial: whether to initiate early to give maximum clinical benefit or later to minimise motor side-effects. Generally it is acceptable to start treatment when difficulty managing activities of daily living is encountered. Low-dose L-dopa three times a day is a common starting regimen and remains the gold standard despite the range of drug treatment now available.

More clinicians are now using dopamine agonists as early monotherapy (particularly in younger patients) as well as adjunct therapy later on. COMT inhibitors are used as adjunct therapy earlier rather than later on. Apomorphine is helpful in severely fluctuating/freezing patients. Combined therapy is commonly started early on in the disease process.

Long-term adverse effects of anti-parkinsonian drugs (Table 2)

Although L-dopa is initially very helpful in PD, its effects become less apparent with prolonged use as patients become more susceptible to side-effects.

Involuntary movements (dyskinesia) can be caused by the drug and about half of all patients will experience these side-effects within five years of starting treatment. Psychiatric side-effects are also common; patients may experience nightmares, hallucinations, anxiety, depression and/or confusion.

THINKING POINT

- **Effective control of drug regimen is an important component of Parkinson's disease management. What factors need to be taken into account when helping a person with Parkinson's disease manage their medication?**

PART TWO

The role of the nurse

Treatment of Parkinson's disease is concerned with establishing an effective drug programme (Fig 3) and limiting drug side-effects while promoting independence in activities of daily living. The plan of treatment for each patient must be determined on an individual basis as response to treatment varies. Some patients do not need drug intervention in the initial stages as their symptoms are mild; others require extensive regimens.

EMOTIONAL AND PSYCHOLOGICAL SUPPORT

The impact of being told that he or she has a chronic and debilitating condition may cause severe stress for the patient, as well as for his or her family. The acceptance of a diagnosis can follow a similar pattern of shock, disbelief, denial and acceptance as that seen in bereavement. No one wishes to become ill or to learn that they have a

Fig 3. The actions of drug groups in Parkinson's disease

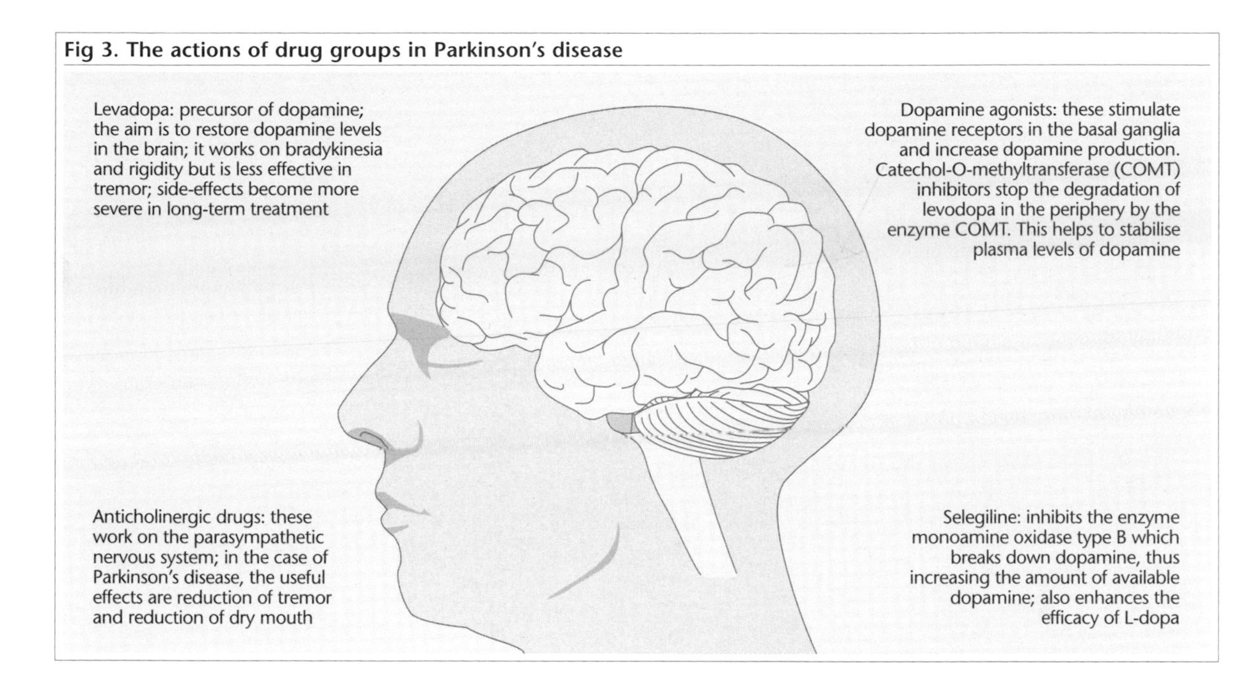

chronic condition that may get worse and for which they will need to take regular medication for the rest of their life.

Some patients express resentment and find it difficult to accept their diagnosis. If this occurs, it is often useful to seek a second opinion. However, denial can persist and severely hamper progress.

Sometimes, the news provokes feelings of anger. Very often, people are near retirement age when they develop PD and, after a lifetime of hard work, they resent the condition because it stops them from going ahead with their retirement plans.

Other patients may immediately see themselves as being chronic invalids, and will express despair and feelings that life is not worth living. Nurses can play a role in helping patients and their families to express the way they are feeling and, when the initial shock has worn off, they can begin to help the patient understand the disorder and the treatment needed to manage it. The patient should be reassured that, although the condition cannot be cured, the symptoms can be controlled and that the aim of the treatment plan will be to foster independence and an active lifestyle.

It is also helpful to explain that, in those with established disease, response to drugs may be variable and may fluctuate throughout the day. Patients may change from being active and responsive to being withdrawn and lethargic within a matter of minutes. Such explanations can help families understand the patient's problems and how best to cope with them. Putting the patient and family in contact with the Parkinson's Disease Society will enable them to access practical advice and information.

ACTIVITIES OF DAILY LIVING

PD, as with most progressive neurological disorders, has a far-reaching effect. Eventually it will have an impact on most areas of a person's life. Activities of daily living are used here as a framework for discussing the effects and the associated nursing care.

Depression

Up to 40% of patients with PD become depressed (Cummings, 1992). This can be a feature of the condition itself or can be a reaction to increased physical difficulties as the disease progresses. Loss of drive and energy caused by depression adds to the inability to cope with daily living and results in fatigue and apathy. It may be difficult to tell whether a patient with PD is actually depressed or just appears that way; reduced facial expression and a monotonous voice are features of both depression and of PD. Antidepressant therapy may in some cases make parkinsonian symptoms worse. This needs to be explained when drugs are prescribed.

Family members may become resentful or irritated by apparent loss of initiative in the patient. The nurse can help by facilitating discussions and openness among members of the family and being aware that these situations and feelings are common. He or she can explain that patients will often appear lethargic and uninterested as a result of the disease process and that this appearance is outside their control.

Communication

Aspects of PD that impact on communication include its effects on speech, eyesight and writing. The ability to

Fig 4. Pill-rolling tremor

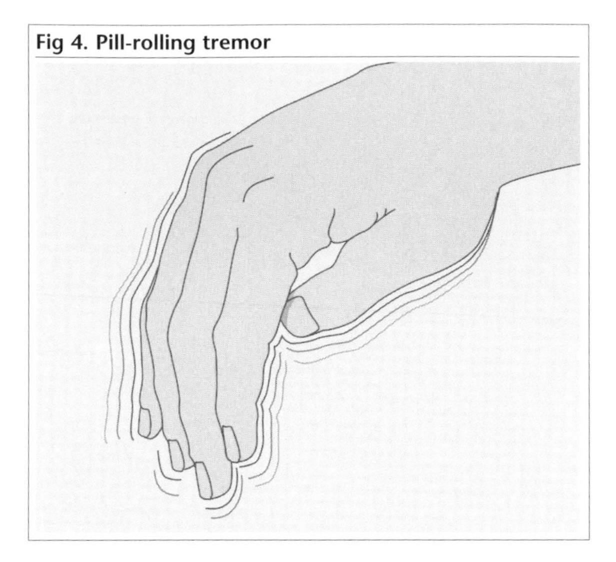

speak requires coordination of the muscles in the larynx and those which deal with breathing and movement around the throat, tongue and nasal passages. Some patients with PD show a reduction in the clarity and volume of speech and have a quiet, monotonous voice (dysphonia).

Such speech difficulties interfere with effective oral communication. If, following assessment, a nurse observes problems in this area, referral to a speech therapy service to provide training in control of the voice and assistance with communication strategies may help. Nurses should take time when dealing with a person who has speech problems, as appearing hurried and exasperated will have a negative impact on their morale.

Patients may have blurred vision caused by anticholinergic drugs which paralyse the eye muscles responsible for constriction of the pupil, resulting in difficulty with reading, sewing or writing.

Occasionally, people with PD have difficulty keeping their eyes open, but this does not necessarily indicate tiredness or fatigue; rather, it is caused by a difficulty with muscle control (Sagar, 1991).

Blinking also occurs less frequently, resulting in a staring expression. This can lead to irritation of the cornea because it is wiped less often by the eyelid. This may be eased by the use of artificial tear preparations.

Micrographia (progressive reduction in the size of handwriting) sometimes develops in PD. The handwriting may start off the normal size and then become progressively smaller and unintelligible. This is particularly problematic for those who enjoy writing or for whom writing is a major component of their work. There may also be difficulties signing cheques or legal documents. Occupational and speech therapy may help in developing alternative communication strategies.

In addition, social services should be able to advise patients and families if there are problems signing documents or cheques.

Elimination

Those with PD may experience slowness in starting to pass urine, dribbling of urine for some time after micturition, and frequency of micturition. These symptoms result from a difficulty in coordinating the muscles that control the bladder but can be exacerbated by anticholinergic drugs.

Urinary problems can also result from a variety of conditions unrelated to PD but which are common in older people. A detailed history should be gathered in order to eliminate the other possibilities such as infection, prolapsed uterus or prostatic enlargement.

Patients can feel embarrassed when discussing continence and nurses should ensure they provide a suitably private environment and approach the issue sensitively . Adopt a positive, reassuring attitude and enlist the help of a continence adviser at an early stage.

Constipation is common among older people, but it can be exacerbated in PD (Calne, 1994). It can occur because the muscles in the bowels become sluggish. Anticholinergic drugs can cause constipation too. When discussing this problem with the patient, nurses should try to establish the person's normal routine and provide advice about the amount of fibre, fresh fruit and vegetables, fluid intake, exercise and sensible use of laxatives.

People with PD are at increased risk of poor nutrition and weight loss because of poor swallowing and dyskinesia. Dietetic involvement and attention to diet are an important part of care.

Loss of finger dexterity (Fig 4)

Patients with mild PD may experience difficulty with tasks such as fastening buttons, threading needles and counting change. With advancement of the disease, the problems may increase to include normal activities associated with washing, dressing and eating. Finger dexterity is one of the most noticeable aspects of movement to be affected by the disease and the ability to move the fingers independently is lost. Nurses can work closely with other members of a multidisciplinary team, particularly occupational therapists, when assessing problems with washing and dressing (Jameson, 1995).

Maintaining a safe environment

In normal health, we have a reflex action that rapidly comes into place to correct the fall in blood pressure that occurs on standing. In PD this reflex is sluggish and there is a tendency to postural hypotension (a fall in blood pressure on standing up). Postural hypotension may also be caused or exacerbated by anti-parkinsonian drugs. If patients with PD complain of dizziness, their blood pressure should be checked lying down, sitting upright and after standing for a minute or two. A fall of more than 20mmHg systolic (or 10mmHg diastolic) on sitting or standing is usually significant. Treatment should be minimised to try to reduce the degree of postural hypotension.

However, many patients with PD will need to take fairly large doses of levadopa (L-dopa) for mobility and this will inevitably cause some postural hypotension. They will have to strike a balance between the beneficial effects of the drugs on their mobility and their adverse effects on blood pressure.

They may find it helpful to use techniques that minimise the risk from postural hypotension. They should be taught not to get up suddenly but, rather, to sit on the edge of the bed for one or two minutes before standing and should stand from a chair slowly. They need to avoid standing for long periods in one place or, if they have to, should regularly transfer their weight from one foot to another. The symptoms increase if the patient is in a hot environment (because of vasodilatation), so this should be avoided. Symptoms can also be controlled by raising the head of the bed by 7–10cm at night and by wearing elastic stockings to support venous return from the legs. Fludrocortisone may also help counteract hypotension.

Sexual function

Many people have difficulty discussing sexual issues. The nurse needs to understand that sexual activity does not stop being important when someone is chronically ill. The nurse is in a prime role to educate the patient in this area and allay unfounded fears. Very often it is claimed that sexual problems in Parkinson's patients arise more from fear of failure than from real physical handicap. If the patient is depressed this may also affect their sex drive. Drugs, such as anticholinergics, can interfere with a man's ability to achieve an erection.

It is important to include sexual function in the overall assessment of a patient's needs. After the elimination of primary causes of dysfunction, practical suggestions (including timing of medication) or discussion of what sex can involve may help. Referral to a specialist either to further eliminate other causes or counselling if the problem continues should be considered. It is essential that the nurse does not trivialise or dismiss concerns that the patient may have in this area.

Mobility

Bradykinesia is a key feature of PD and causes difficulty in initiating activities, especially walking. There is slowness of movement with all activities of daily living, and nurses should allow for this.

Rigidity can also cause problems. There is increased tone in the muscles and this leads to a stooped posture with legs and arms slightly flexed. The combination of bradykinesia and rigidity accounts for the disturbance in posture, gait and dexterity.

Apart from the involuntary tremor, which may not be present, the ability to achieve spontaneous movement is largely lost. The patient may have difficulty getting up from a low chair. If this is the case, he or she may find it easier to use a high-backed chair with arm rests.

There is also a tendency to fall over after standing because of failure to achieve rapid balance in posture and postural hypotension. Once upright, the patient can appear rooted to the spot (akinetic). If this happens, it is useful to employ one of several tactics. Some patients benefit from walking on the spot or singing, clicking fingers or stepping over an imaginary line and then taking a sudden step forward. Others find that starting to count to themselves, setting a target to start walking on six or seven may help. In some cases, it may be helpful to help the patient gain momentum by rocking backwards and forwards before starting to walk.

Normal walking requires an upright posture and a swing of the arms. In advanced cases of PD, the head is thrown downward and arm swing is lost.

Walking takes place with a series of small steps and the chest is often in front of the feet, which alters the centre of gravity. If the feet or foot catch on an object this can rapidly propel the patient forward and he or she will fall. Problems also occur when the patient is required to stop suddenly, change direction or turn. Turning is a particular problem, as the head and body do not move independently, and it has to be accomplished as a whole-body manoeuvre.

Lack of coordination obviously poses a problem for patients when they encounter narrow paths or objects within the normal line of walking, as these interfere with their normal rhythm of walking. They might freeze on the spot or carry out a series of unproductive small steps or lose balance and fall. For this reason, it is essential to work with a physiotherapist and an occupational therapist, as well as the patients and their relatives, to ensure that the home of the person with PD is adapted to make it safe. Visual blocks can occur in doorways. Looking through the doorway may help. This is known as visual cueing.

The nurse should also advise the patient about exercise and its benefits in maintaining supple joints and muscles, in improving physical coordination and posture, in enhancing awareness of body position as well as increasing dexterity in the hands.

The physiotherapist can advise on how to improve and control breathing and teach techniques to improve walking and cope with activities of daily living. This teaching should be reinforced by nurses as part of the overall plan to manage the patient's condition.

In addition to problems related to muscle control and movement, sweating, greasy skin (seborrhoea) and increased salivation are associated with PD. Positioning of the head can also play a part.

Patients may also drool saliva from the corner of the mouth which may be a result of difficulty in normal swallowing, although sometimes PD itself can produce excessive saliva. Explanation of the causes of salivation and sweating may help patients and their families. Encouraging the patient to keep his or her head up, supported by the hand if need be, and to consciously swallow more frequently may help. Sometimes hyocine patches are used to reduce secretions, but can cause confusion. Rarely, radiotherapy to the salivary glands may be considered.

Patients may be admitted to hospital for drug adjustment or because their condition is worsening and they can no longer manage independently at home. Following hospital admission of a patient with advanced or moderate PD, nurses need to recognise the connection between drugs and mobility.

Drug programmes to help control the symptoms of PD are individual and therefore drug times differ from those of the standard drug rounds. Patients cannot wait for their drugs and need to be given them at the exact time of the prescription. It may be appropriate to maintain a chart, detailing the effects of the drugs on mobility. It is better if patients keep their own mobility chart. These are known as 'on-off' charts and involve marking half-hourly boxes to indicate whether he or she is 'on' — able to mobilise; 'on with dyskinesia' — able to mobilise but with involuntary movements; or 'off' — unable to mobilise effectively. In the light of this information, drug regimen/doses or daily activity timings can be adjusted to optimise the patient's day and night.

Nursing patients with PD can be challenging — especially if patients are known over many years. Initially, the onset of PD may be gradual with few symptoms. As the disease progresses, the level of intervention from healthcare professionals will increase.

The nurse has a key role, both in the hospital and in the community setting, in helping patients and their relatives understand and control symptoms of the disease in order to maintain maximum independence.

THINKING POINT

- **Think about people with Parkinson's disease for whom you have cared. How successful were you in helping them with communication difficulties? How might you approach these problems differently?**

PART THREE

Revision notes

Parkinson's disease is a disorder of voluntary movement caused by deficiency of a neurotransmitter called dopamine in the substantia nigra of the brain (Fig 5). This is responsible for the clinical presentation of PD and is the rationale for drug treatment. Standard treatment aims to raise the level of dopamine in the substantia nigra by giving levadopa (L-dopa), which is a precursor of dopamine; it is converted to dopamine when it enters the brain. In the UK, the most recent estimates of overall prevalence of PD are 140–160 per 100,000 of population.

The cause of the disease is unknown. Genetic factors do not seem to be important, neither is there satisfactory

Fig 5. The action of dopamine working as a neurotransmitter in the brain

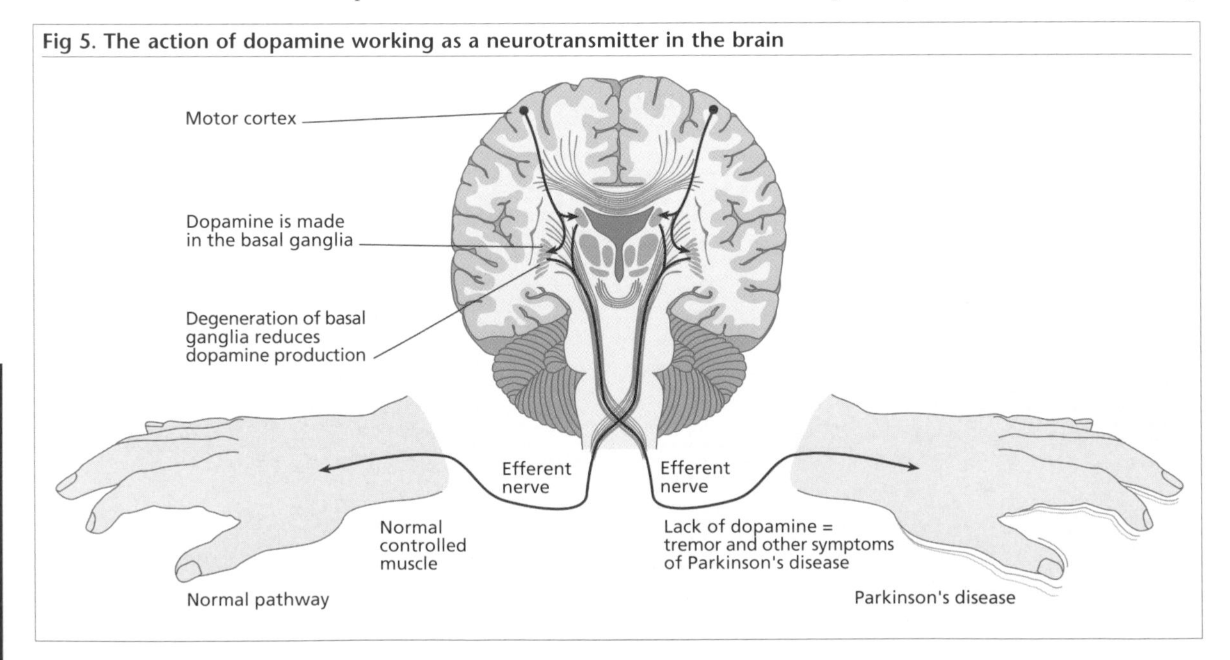

evidence of a viral cause. Hereditary factors, although originally discounted, have recently emerged as a focus of PD research (Polymeropoulos, 1998).

A wide variety of agents have been considered from infectious, toxic and other exposures. It is now known that non-smokers have a greater risk of disease although the reason for this is unclear (Birtwistle and Hall, 1996). People exposed to pesticides and with head injury also show a consistently elevated risk but are prone to biased measurement. It is likely that the cause is multifactorial, with contributions of variable significance from genetic predisposition, environmental toxins and ageing.

To make a diagnosis, it is necessary to identify bradykinesia plus one other key feature. The key features that substantiate a Parkinson's diagnosis are:

- Bradykinesia: slowness of movement and a difficulty in starting movement
- Rigidity: the presence of increased tone in the muscles, leading to a characteristic stooped posture and flexed limbs
- Postural instability: this comes as a result of poor muscular control; people with PD are at risk of falling over
- Tremor: this comes as a result of poor control over fine muscle movement; known as 'pill rolling' or resting tremor (Fig 4) is characteristic of the disease, but tremor alone is not a basis for diagnosis.

Some associated minor features may also be present. These are:

- Seborrhoea or excessive sweating
- Dysphonia: people with PD may experience difficulty with speaking
- Dysphagia: difficulty with swallowing can mean a risk of inhalation of food or liquid, and chest infection as the disease progresses
- Excessive salivation
- Forward flexion of the spine
- Micrographia: a phenomenon in which the patient's handwriting becomes progressively smaller
- Depression
- Anxiety
- Mild to moderate dementia.

While tremor is quite often present, it is not of itself essential for a diagnosis and many patients (particularly older people) have tremor that is not related to PD.

PARKINSONISM

Several other conditions can mimic PD but the underlying pathological processes are different. Parkinsonism is a term used to describe the symptoms of PD, which can be divided into four categories:

- Primary or idiopathic: PD
- Secondary: drug-induced (due to neuroleptics, some antiemetics, MPTP) trauma, stroke, tumour
- Parkinson's-plus syndromes, for example multiple system atrophy, progressive supranuclear palsy, Shy Drager syndrome, Lewy body disease
- Hereditary degenerative disease, for example, Huntington's disease, Wilson's disease

DRUG TREATMENT

The main types of drugs used in the treatment of PD are:

- Levadopa: L-dopa is a precursor of dopamine; dopamine cannot be given directly as it does not cross the blood–brain barrier. Preparations include co-careldopa and co-beneldopa
- Dopamine agonists: these are drugs which increase levels of dopamine; for example, bromocriptine, pergolide, lysuride and apomorphine
- Selegiline: this is a selective inhibitors of an enzyme that breaks down dopamine and is thought to delay progression of the disease
- Anticholinergics: for example, benzhexol, which reduce tremor and can be used to help excessive salivation.
- Catechol-O-methyltransferase (COMT) inhibitors: these agents inhibit the degradation of levodopa through the enzyme catechol-O-methyltransferase. They were launched in 1998. Tolcapone was withdrawn in late 1998 and entacapone is now the only one available on the UK market.

Side-effects

None of the drugs used in the treatment of PD are without their adverse affects. L-dopa preparations can cause nausea and should be taken on a full stomach.

They can also cause postural hypotension which, combined with existing unsteadiness, increases the risk of falls. Other side-effects include sweating attacks and confusion.

Although L-dopa is initially very helpful in PD, its effects become less apparent with prolonged use as patients become more susceptible to side-effects.

Involuntary movements (dyskinesia) can be caused by the drug and about half of all patients will experience these within five years of starting treatment. Psychiatric side-effects are also common; patients may experience nightmares, hallucinations, anxiety, depression or confusion.

Using high levels of L-dopa to achieve absence of symptoms of PD produces these side-effects but several drugs can modify the response. As the disease progresses polypharmacy becomes inevitable. Dopamine agonists and COMT inhibitors may be valuable in avoiding long-term consequences of L-dopa for some patients as they keep the overall doses of L-dopa lower for longer.

Dopamine agonist drugs such as bromocriptine can also cause nausea. Once again this may be helped by giving the drug with food. Like L-dopa, it can also cause hypotension and longer-term psychological effects.

Anticholinergic drugs can cause dry mouth (which can sometimes be helpful in PD), constipation and urinary retention.

Drug prescription is a skilled job requiring regular review. Adherence to the drug regimen is important (MacSweeney, 1992). Hospital admission can disrupt a patient's normal drug therapy, thus nurses must be careful to keep as closely as possible to the patient's normal regimen.

CASE HISTORIES

Onset of PD is insidious and the diagnosis may be unclear for up to a year or two. At this stage patients may mistakenly be thought to have had a stroke or arthritic complaints, particularly if, as commonly occurs, the onset is more marked on one side of the body than the other.

Some patients may be thought to have depression or early dementia. Patients may think the diagnosis unlikely if tremor is not present and others may worry that tremors caused by other conditions are due to Parkinson's.

Many patients may be concerned about developing dementia, which is known to occur in PD. It effects about 20% of patients, with a higher prevalence in the older patient (Water, 1998).

Parkinson's dementia is subcortical. It is differentiated from cortical dementia (Alzheimer's) by a syndrome of slow cortical responses, memory loss and poor concentration/initiative. All reversible causes of dementia, such as vitamin B12 deficiency, hypothyroidism, lesions, neurosyphyllis and hydrocephalus, must be eliminated. Diffuse Lewy body disease is similar to Alzheimer's and is the extreme spectrum of PD.

Early Parkinson's disease: case study

Daniel Partridge is 66 years old and has not been well since he retired from his job as a bank clerk last year. He had intended to have an active retirement but now has gradually stopped going to see friends and has neglected his allotment.

He seems less motivated and on a couple of occasions has unexpectedly fallen over at home. He has been particularly clumsy using his left hand recently.

His wife says that he is rather withdrawn and does not smile very much; she thinks that he may be depressed. She eventually insists that he see the doctor when she notices that he has started keeping his left hand under the newspaper when they have visitors because he has developed a tremor.

● Comment: It is most likely that Mr Partridge has early Parkinson's with onset on the left side. Patients may hide a limb affected by tremor because of embarrassment about the disorder. Depression is a feature of the disease, but patients may only appear to be unhappy because of the effects of Parkinson's on the facial muscles.

Established Parkinson's disease: case study

Elizabeth Drury is 72 and has had PD for seven years. She has been treated with co-careldopa, one tablet five times per day and selegiline 10mg in the morning.

She had been admitted to hospital following a fall when she sustained a fractured neck of femur. The surgery for this went well, but she has still not started to mobilise one week later. She has only been written up for three co-careldopa tablets per day, although she eventually manages to get this changed.

She is thought to be a bit awkward by ward staff because she always asks for her drugs at times when they are busy and never seems to want them at the times of the normal drug rounds. The physiotherapist thinks she is difficult as well because on some occasions she seems to be able to mobilise very well then, just a few minutes later, insists that she cannot walk at all.

● Comment: Patients with established disease treated with L-dopa preparations are often very sensitive to small changes in dosages and timing of drugs. Patients usually know when they need their drugs and what dose they should have.

Medical and nursing staff, particularly those in wards not used to Parkinson's patients, may not fully appreciate this. These patients are also prone to severe fluctuations in their mobility (the 'on/off' effect), which might be misunderstood by some staff.

NURSING INTERVENTIONS

Nurses need to work with medical staff and therapists and other members of a multidisciplinary team when managing patients with PD.They need to consider:

● Communication, both spoken and written

● Mobility: consideration of problems in initiating and maintaining mobility; transfers and bed mobility (Fig 6)

● Elimination: control of bladder and bowel; attention to constipation; diet

● Medication: individual dose schedules for drugs; attention to possible side-effects

● Swallowing and diet

● Personal hygiene: washing, dressing and toileting

● Psychological problems: depression and confusion.

Professionals from other disciplines will often be able to help in the management of patients with PD and nurses should consider appropriate referral, for example:

● Physiotherapy: can help with mobility and transfers, walking aids and advice (for example, on techniques to reduce the risks from postural hypotension)

● Occupational therapy: assessment and advice on washing, dressing and toileting; appropriate adaptations and appliances

● Speech and language therapy: can help with swallowing problems and communication difficulties; strategies for overcoming these

● Dietetics: dietary advice in the light of possible swallowing problems, constipation, reduced mobility and the adverse effects of some drugs

● Clinical psychology: assessment of cognitive deficits and depressive symptoms; counselling

● Continence adviser: assessment and management of continence problems

Fig 6. Using exaggerated movements to start walking

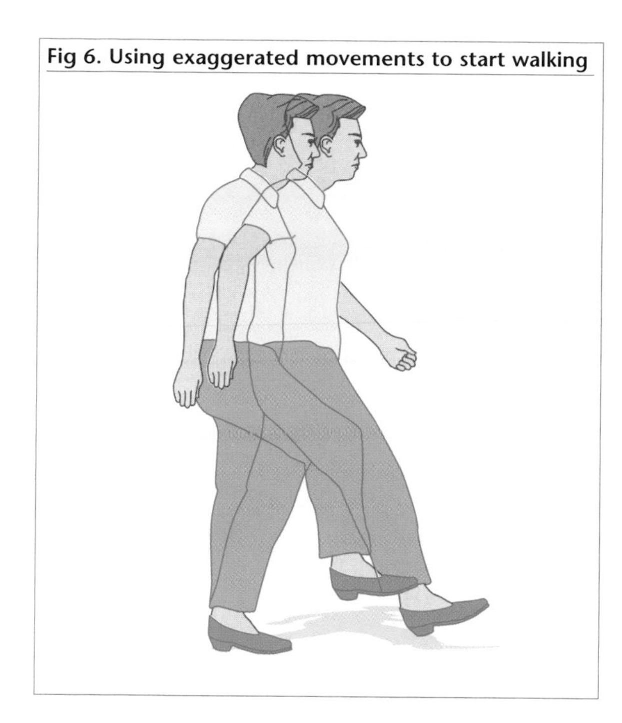

- Social work: financial and benefits advice, community care assessment.

EMOTIONAL SUPPORT

Chronic illness is stressful for both the patient and carers. Frequently people are around retirement age when they develop PD and, after a life-time of hard work, they resent the condition as it stops them from going ahead with their retirement plans.

Once the initial shock of diagnosis has worn off, nurses can begin to help the patient understand the disorder and the treatment needed.

It is also helpful to explain that, in those with established disease, response to drugs may fluctuate throughout the day; patients can change from being active and responsive to being withdrawn and lethargic within a matter of minutes.

Knowing this can help families understand the patient's problems and how best to cope with them. Support groups such as the Parkinson's Disease Society provide access to practical information.

ADVANCES IN TREATMENT

Recently a document called *Parkinson's Aware in Primary Care* was sent to all GPs in the UK. Based on a four-stage framework, it is a new paradigm for medical and nursing priorities during the disease progression.

It emphasises consistent management and planning right from the start as a team to help deliver better care, cost-effectively to the person with PD and his or her family. Using this combined approach as a model, the short- and long-term aims and nursing management of PD can be assessed.

REFERENCES

Ben-Shlomo, Y. (1997) The epidemiology of Parkinson's disease. *Ballieres Clinical Neurology*; 6: 1, 5548.

Birtwistle, J., Hall, K. (1996) Does nicotine have beneficial effects in the treatment of certain diseases? *British Journal of Nursing* 5: 19: 1195–1202.

Calne, S. (1994) Nursing care of patients with ideopathic Parkinson's disease. *Nursing Times*; 90: 24, 38.

Cummings, J.L. (1992) Depression and Parkinson's disease. *American Journal of Psychiatry*; 194: 4, 443–453.

Jameson, M. (1995) Helping new patients with Parkinson's. *Care of the Elderly*; 17: 2, 193–205.

MacMahon, D. (1990) Parkinson's disease in context. *Care of the Elderly*; 2: 1, 4–8.

MacMahon, D., Thomas, S. (1998) Practical approach to quality of life in Parkinson's disease: the nurse's role. *Journal of Neurology*; 245: suppl 1, S19–22.

MacSweeney, J. (1992) A helpful assessment medication regime of one patient with Parkinson's disease. *Nursing Times* 1992; 88: 29, 32–33.

Polymeropoulos, M.H. ((1998) Autosomal dominant Parkinson's disease and alpha-synclein. *Annals of Neurology*; 44: suppl 1, S63–64.

Quinn, N. (1995) Drug treatment of Parkinson's disease. *British Medical Journal* 1995; 310: 575–579.

Roberts, G.W. et al (1993) *Neuropsychiatric Disorders*. London: Wolfe Publishing.

Sagar, H. (1991) *Parkinson's Disease: Positive Health Guide*. London: Macdonald Optima.

FURTHER READING

Barker, E. (1992) *Neuroscience Nursing*. St Louis, Missouri: Mosby Year Book.

Bunting. L.K., Fitzsimmons, B. (1991) Depression in Parkinson's disease. *Journal of Neuroscience Nursing*; 23: 3, 158–164.

Fitzsimmons, B., Bunting, L.K. (1993) Parkinson's disease: quality of life issues. *Neuroscience Nursing*; 28: 4, 807–818.

Hickey, J.V. (1992) *The Clinical Practice of Neurological and Neurosurgical Nursing*. Philadelphia, Penn: Lippincott.

Kelly, G. (1995) A self-care approach . . . Parkinson's disease. *Nursing Times*; 91: 2, 40–41.

Peace, G. (1995) Living with Parkinson's disease. *Nursing Times*; 91: 32, 40–41.

Useful addresses

Parkinson's Disease Society, 215 Vauxhall Bridge Road, London SW1V 1EJ. Tel: 0171 931 8080. Helpline: 0171 233 5373

Sexual Problems of the Disabled (SPOD), 286 Camden Road, London N7 0BJ. Tel: 0171 607 8851

Disabled Living Foundation, 380 Harrow Road, London W9. Tel: 0171 289 6111

Carers National Association, 29 Chilworth Mews, London WC 3RJ. Tel: 0171 490 8818

Parkinson's disease

Assessment

When you have read the unit and completed any further reading, you can use the questions below to test your understanding of the topic. Answers can be found on the next page.

1 PD may be due to:

1. Dopamine deficiency in the substantia nigra
2. Drugs such as haloperidol
3. Recurrent strokes
4. All of the above

2 Postural hypotension:

1. Is uncommon in PD
2. Rarely does any harm
3. Can be made worse by levadopa
4. Cannot be treated

3 Patients with PD:

1. Never develop dementia
2. Are nearly always depressed
3. Can develop problems with handwriting
4. Get dry skin

4 Levadopa preparations:

1. Cause dry mouth
2. Are not often used nowadays
3. Can cause involuntary movements
4. Can only be given by injection

5 Drug treatment of PD:

1. Is the same for all patients
2. Usually consists of anticholinergic drugs
3. Usually only needs to be given once a day
4. Can cause the on/off effect

6 Nurses can help patients with PD by:

1. Restricting their mobility in case they fall
2. Asking the doctor to increase their drugs if they are confused
3. Washing and dressing them to save them embarrassment if they are too slow
4. Teaching them strategies to overcome postural hypotension

7 Onset of PD:

1. Is usually obvious
2. Is probably the cause of most tremors in old people
3. Can be mistaken for a stroke
4. Occurs suddenly

8 Parkinsonism, a term used to describe the symptoms of PD:

1. Mimics PD
2. Can be caused by temazepam
3. Can be related to recurrent strokes
4. All of the above

9 In the treatment of PD

1. Some drugs have to be given by injection
2. Surgery is commonly used
3. Drugs rarely causes side-effects
4. Treatment works best in advanced disease

10 In PD tremor is:

1. Never a symptom
2. Always a symptom
3. Frequently a symptom
4. Worse on activity

11 Patients with PD can experience micrographia, which is:

1. A progressive reduction in the size of hand writing
2. Inability to open the eyelids
3. An increase in the size of handwriting
4. An inability to blink normally

12 A typical complaint related to passing urine is:

1. Urgency in passing urine
2. Frequent urinary tract infections
3. Retention of urine
4. Slowness in starting to pass urine

13 **Following the news that a patient has been diagnosed as having PD you should:**

- [ ] 1 Contact a religious representative for reassurance
- [ ] 2 Tell the patient that everything will be OK
- [ ] 3 Provide as much accurate information about the condition as you can
- [ ] 4 Refuse to answer any more questions before talking to the doctor involved

14 **In PD:**

- [ ] 1 Patients may appear depressed, and true depression is common
- [ ] 2 Depression usually responds to advice such as: 'Pull yourself together'
- [ ] 3 Depression may be difficult to detect
- [ ] 4 Depression occurs only late in the disease

15 **Levodopa preparation causes less nausea if taken:**

- [ ] 1 On an empty stomach
- [ ] 2 With fluids only
- [ ] 3 On a full stomach
- [ ] 4 In the night

16 **PD occurs:**

- [ ] 1 At any time
- [ ] 2 Can occur in the young, but it usually occurs in people over the age of 50
- [ ] 3 Only over 50 years of age
- [ ] 4 More frequently in women than in men

ANSWERS

Parkinson's disease

1: PD may be due to:
4) All of the above

2: Postural hypotension:
3) Can be made worse by levadopa

3: Patients with PD:
4) All of the above

4: Levadopa preparations:
1) Cause dry mouth

5: Drug treatment of PD:
4) Can cause the on/off effect

6: Nurses can help patients with PD by:
4) Teaching them strategies to overcome postural hypotension

7: Onset of PD:
3) Can be mistaken for a stroke

8: Parkinsonism, a term used to describe the symptoms of PD:
1) All of the above

9: In the treatment of PD
1) Some drugs have to be given by injection

10: In PD tremor is:
3) Frequently a symptom

11: Patients with PD can experience micrographia, which is:
1) A progressive reduction in the size of handwriting

12: A typical complaint related to passing urine is:
4) Slowness in starting to pass urine

13: Following the news that a patient has been diagnosed as having PD, you should:
3) Provide as much accurate information about the condition as you can

14: In PD:
1) Patients may appear depressed, and true depression is common

15: Levodopa preparation causes less nausea if taken:
3) On a full stomach

16: PD occurs:
2) Can occur in the young but usually occurs in people over the age of 50

Stroke

Knowledge for practice

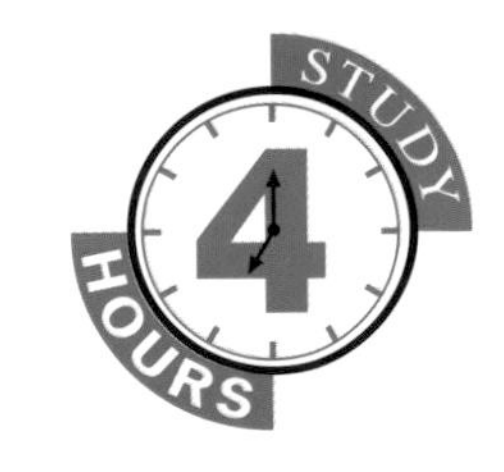

One of the greatest challenges in nursing lies in the care of people who have had a stroke, but it is also one of the most rewarding. Stroke, as a medical condition, is easy to understand, but its effects are not, being different in every case to a greater or lesser degree. It is in the individualisation of a patient's care that the challenge lies, because, while the treatment of a stroke's physical effects may be relatively straightforward, the psychological effects can be difficult to understand, let alone to deal with.

For stroke treatment to have any chance of success, a team approach must be used. With the exception of the patient and his family, no individual in the team is more of less important than any other. Perhaps this is best described as a 'supradisciplinary' approach, rather than multi- or interdisciplinary, both of which suggest that there are definite boundaries between the professions which should not be crossed.

However, nursing occupies a distinct place in the overall picture of stroke care, as nurses are the only practitioners to have 24-hour contact with patients. For this reason, within specialised stroke units, while overall responsibility for care may lie with a physician or geriatrician, it is likely that the role of coordinator will fall naturally upon a nurse or group of nurses.

In some units, the coordinator may be a physiotherapist or, more rarely, an occupational therapist. Provided that there are good lines of communication, commitment to team working on the part of all the professionals involved and consistency in the delivery of planned care, the primary qualification of the person assuming this role is probably unimportant.

EPIDEMIOLOGY

A campaign launched at the end of 1995 by the Stroke Association aimed to inform the public about how widespread stroke is, with the message 'every five minutes, someone has a stroke'. After cancer and cardiovascular disease, stroke is the third largest cause of death in the UK (Swaffield, 1990). More significantly perhaps, it is the condition that most commonly causes disability throughout the whole of the Western world (King, 1990).

As stroke treatment is continuously being refined and improved, with more specialised units being established all the time, stroke is unlikely to lose its leading place in this grim league table.

ANATOMY AND PHYSIOLOGY OF STROKE

A stroke occurs when there is a sudden disruption in the supply of blood to the brain and cells are affected by the disruption in the supply of oxygen. The disruption can be caused by thrombosis, embolism or haemorrhage. A thrombus is a blood clot, formed within the circulation, which remains stationary. If thrombi become large enough, the vessel may be occluded. An embolus, on the other hand, is anything carried in the circulation which can block off blood vessels, such as a thrombus which has become detached, air bubbles or the plaque formed in atherosclerosis. Brain cells are particularly sensitive to changes in oxygenation, and infarction can set in within minutes, with no hope of regeneration in the cells (Fig 1).

Fig 1. Mechanism of stroke: cerebral infarction

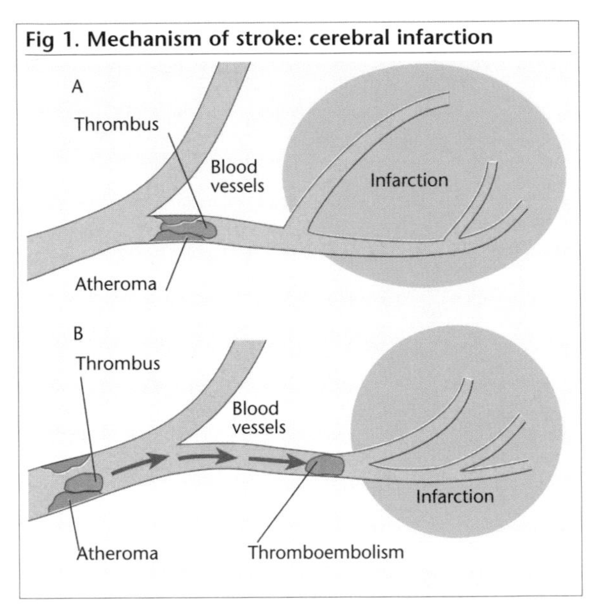

Strokes are often called cerebrovascular accidents or CVAs. Some practitioners may talk about 'mini-strokes', or transient ischaemic attacks (TIAs) if the symptoms are not long-lasting or are not particularly severe.

This can be misleading; in fact, the distinction between a CVA and a TIA is quite clear in the definition provided by the World Health Organization (WHO). If signs and symptoms disappear before 24 hours elapse, then it is a TIA, irrespective of their severity; but if they persist beyond the 24-hour marker, it is a CVA (WHO, 1971).

The WHO definition includes subarachnoid haemorrhage as a cause of stroke but excludes subdural haematoma and damage (including haemorrhage) caused by infections or neoplasms; the apparent primary cause of the event must be vascular in origin.

Another important distinction is between the 'stroke in evolution' and the 'complete stroke'. In the former, there is a growing area of cerebral infarction, which results in neurological deficits that worsen over 24-48 hours; a completed stroke is one in which the area of damage is stable in size. The neurological deficits associated with completed stroke can vary enormously.

Signs and symptoms of particular importance are:

- Hemiplegia (complete paralysis of one side of the body)
- Hemiparesis (one-sided weakness)
- Aphasia (speech disturbances)
- Sensory problems (especially visual).

Cerebral blood supply (Fig 2)

Oxygenated blood is delivered to the brain by the four vessels: the two internal carotid arteries and two vertebral arteries. From these, progressively smaller vessels arise to carry blood to all parts of the brain.

These four arteries are connected by the circle of Willis, or circulus arteriosus, at the base of the brain. This vitally important junction is, in the average adult, about three centimetres in diameter.

It should be remembered that the skull has almost no elasticity. So, if there is any bleeding or swelling within the skull cavity, pressure will be exerted on all surrounding areas.

Aetiology of stroke

Of the three main causes of disruption to cerebral blood supply leading to stroke, thrombosis is most common, followed by embolism; haemorrhagic stroke is the least common (Fig 3). Atherosclerosis, a form of arteriosclerosis, is probably the most important contributory factor. Blood does not normally clot within the circulatory system, because the lining of vessels is made up of smooth tissue (the tunica intima). The walls of an atherosclerotic vessel, however, are less smooth and elastic; and, as the condition progresses, the probability of clot formation rises.

Once a clot has formed, it will tend to grow comparatively rapidly, forming a thrombus which can completely occlude the vessel; or the clot may break away, becoming an embolus which will travel along the arterial system's ever smaller vessels until it lodges where the vessel lumen is too narrow for it to pass through intact. The hardened deposits on the atherosclerotic artery walls can also break off and become emboli, with the same result.

While the risk of thrombosis rises with age, cerebral haemorrhage can affect anyone at any time. Most commonly, the bleeding starts at a weak spot — an aneurysm: being under constant pressure from the pumping of blood around the system, these tend to become thinner as they stretch.

An analogy is to think of an inner tube bulging through a tear in a bicycle tyre wall (Booth, 1994). Should pressure increase past the point which the system can safely absorb, the aneurysm may start to leak or burst instantly.

Anything which adversely affects the smooth operation of the arterial system will increase the risk of stroke. Everyone's arteries harden over time, but this does not mean that strokes are an inevitable outcome of ageing; there is much truth in the saying 'a person is as old as his (or her) arteries'. Hypertension, obesity, diabetes mellitus and cigarette smoking have all been singled out as important risk factors. Risk factors for stroke has been divided into five groups by two UK epidemiologists:

- Biological traits that cannot be altered (age, sex)
- Physiological characteristics with high predictive ability, such as blood pressure, serum cholesterol, body mass index
- Behaviours that may be related to other stroke risk factors or could increase risk through mechanisms as yet unknown; for example, poor diet, smoking and alcohol misuse
- Social characteristics such a social class or ethnicity, which show different degrees of risk, although the reasons may not be clear
- Environmental features, which can be biological, psychosocial or physical (Marmot and Poulter, 1992).

The permutations of these risk factors make it unlikely that a single characteristic of the individual can be pinned down as explaining why he or she has succumbed to stroke; it is probably the complex interplay of a number of them which determines why X becomes a stroke victim

Fig 2. Cerebral blood supply

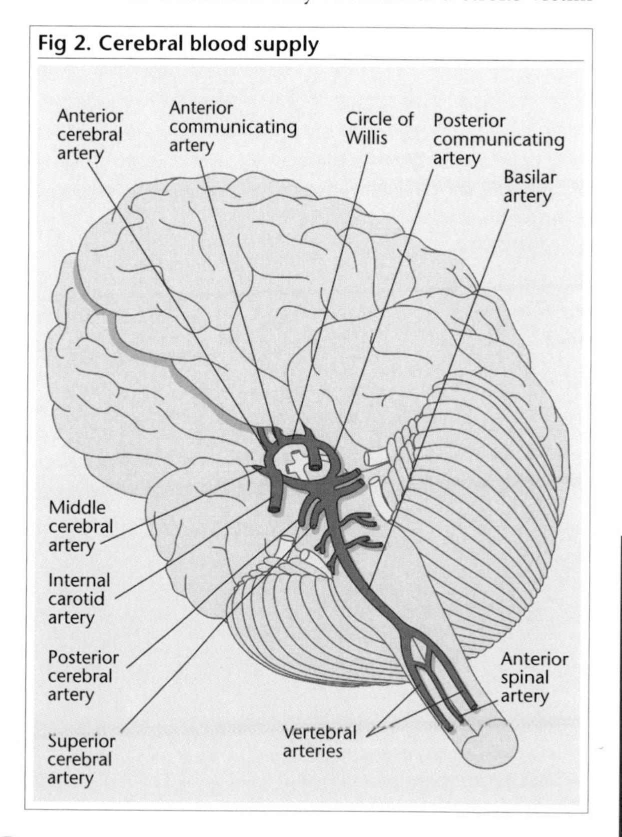

STROKE

after following a healthy lifestyle for years, while Y who exists on junk food and nicotine does not.

DIAGNOSIS

Diagnosis of stroke is made by clinical observation of signs and symptoms and the ruling out of possible alternative explanations. In the UK, sophisticated imaging systems such as computerised axial tomography (CT scanning) and magnetic resonance imaging are most often used to confirm a diagnosis.

There is no such thing as a 'typical' stroke, except in the crudest description of clinical signs. Because the brain is so compact, some of the effects of a stroke in one site can be very different to those that would have been seen had it happened a few millimetres away. The size of the area affected is also critical.

The location of the stroke can be roughly determined, in many cases, by interpretation of signs and symptoms (Fig 4):

- The left hemisphere of the brain controls the opposite side of the body, and vice versa, so 'a left CVA' would be one affecting the right-hand side of the body.
- Because the part of the brain controlling speech is usually in the left hemisphere, a left CVA might affected the ability to speak and understand what is being said.
- If the middle cerebral artery is affected, there may be aphasia, disturbances in the visual field and weakness on the affected side more severe in the arm than the leg.
- If the carotid artery is affected, paralysis and numbness on the affected side will occur, together with changes in sensory perception, lowered level of consciousness and aphasia.
- If the vertebrobasilar artery is affected, hemiparesis, loss of sensation in the lips and mouth, double vision, swallowing the difficulties and memory loss may occur.
- Where the anterior cerebral artery is involved there may be mental disturbances, hemiparesis affecting the leg more than the arm and personality changes.

Fig 3. Mechanism of stroke: cerebral haemorrhage

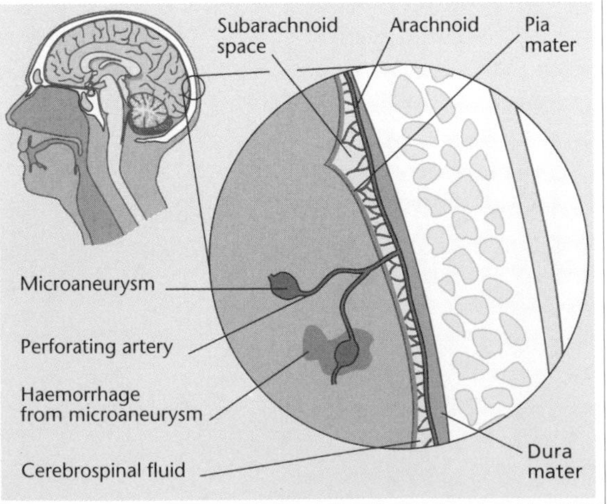

An event affecting the posterior cerebral artery may not result in paralysis, but there is likely to be difficulty in understanding the written word. Part of the visual field may be lost or there may be complete blindness.

PROGNOSIS

Clinicians can only work with the stroke victim's natural rate of recovery. In the best-equipped sites, the chances of the patient receiving rapid and effective treatment for medical emergencies is higher than in other areas, increasing the likelihood of survival; but recovery can only be managed, never accelerated.

In the immediate period following a stroke, any estimates of the patient's likely degree of recovery are just that — estimates; many clinicians will hold their counsel for days or weeks before committing themselves to an opinion. There is a lot of disagreement about the period after which symptoms are likely to continue improving (assuming that they have not disappeared) with different authorities claiming, for example, that the cut-off point lies at three months, six months or a year (Andrews, 1987).

There are some things, though, that seem to hold true for most people who have experienced a stroke:

- The sooner treatment starts, the better the chance of recovery
- The better motivated someone is to recover, the more likely that they will get over their stroke
- Use of an affected leg usually returns before use of the arm, and fine hand movements may take longest of all to recover
- Older memories and skills come back before more recently acquired ones.

TREATMENT

Good nursing care of the stroke patient is made up of lots of small elements and few 'high-tech' major interventions. This is discussed in depth in part two; the following is merely a summary of major areas.

It is worth remembering that a diagnosis of stroke will not automatically lead to hospital admission. Some clinicians believe that the best place to be nursed is at home. Such an approach is dependent, first, on a sound assessment of immediate prognosis and, second, on adequate community support being available. Unsurprisingly, this is an area that has caused considerable debate.

In the initial stages, the first concern is ensuring the patient's safety, particularly if he or she is unconscious, but rehabilitation starts right at the beginning. As in any area of care, assessment is a priority. There are several tools for assessing physical function and psychological status, which gives all-important baseline information.

Spasticity is a word feared in stroke rehabilitation. All joints are controlled by two opposing sets of muscles, one of which flexes the joint, while the other extends it. The flexor muscles are always dominant; to demonstrate this,

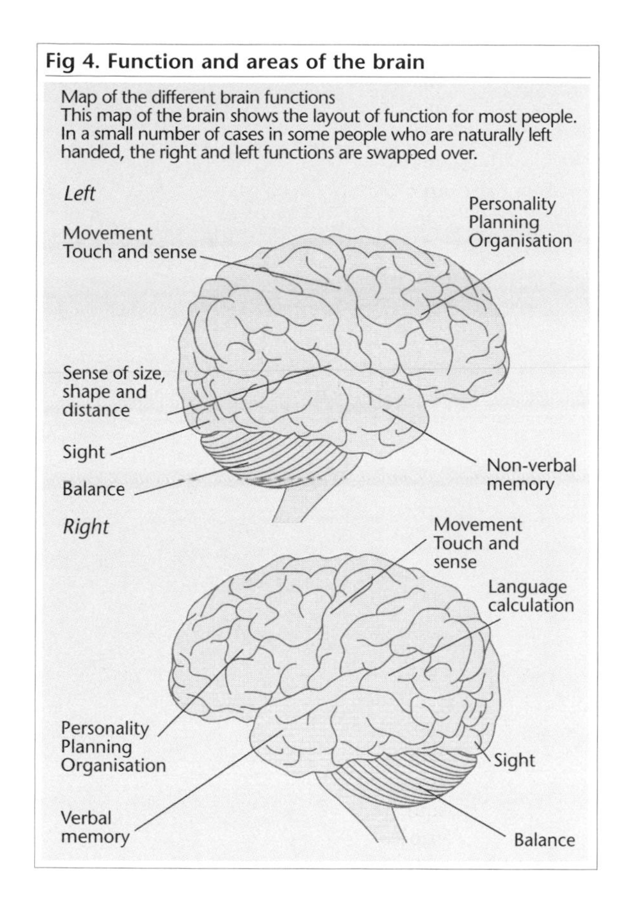

Fig 4. Function and areas of the brain

lay your hands, palm up, on a table and let it relax. Its 'natural' position is not flat but flexed.

After a stroke the muscles on the affected side lose their tone or tension and become flaccid. After a while, tone returns, but it does not stop when normal tonicity is reached; instead, it continues to increase, leading to spasticity. Unchecked, the affected limbs become very contracted; the arm is drawn into the chest, resulting in the classic 'newspaper vendor's posture'. The key to avoiding spasticity lies in correct positioning.

Neglect

Neglect is one of the most unusual phenomena in stroke. It is easy to understand that, when a person has no sensation at all in a part of the body, it can be forgotten; for the person who has had a stroke being able to see the affected limb may make no difference whatsoever. Oliver Sacks, a neurologist, describes 'the man who fell out of bed'. A young man with hemiplegia woke up in hospital, deeply distressed, believing that someone had put a severed human leg into his bed as he slept, and no one could convince him that the leg was his own (Sacks, 1986). When neglect is present, every opportunity must be taken to ensure that the person remains aware of the affected side.

Psychological changes frequently accompany stroke, ranging from short-lived depression to extreme personality changes. Even minor strokes leave patients tired and, with a decrease in functional ability, which may not always be restored, he or she has an uphill struggle ahead. Identification of areas to be treated, and rapid implementation of treatment strategies, is essential. If an individual is to have the best chances of overcoming the problems caused by stroke, care must be individualised, responsive, consistent and based on a sound foundation of accurate knowledge.

THINKING POINTS

- **What is the difference between a transient ischaemic attack and a stroke?**
- **What causes a stroke and what are the risk factors involved?**
- **What kind of feelings do you have when caring for someone who has had a stroke?**

PART TWO

The role of the nurse

Stroke patients occupy 12% of general medical beds. This amounts to a total of around 16000 beds occupied in any one day by stroke patients (Hedley, 1994). Although a number of specialist stroke units have been set up throughout the country, most hospitalised stroke survivors are still occupying beds in wards not specifically geared towards their long-term rehabilitation. Because the incidence of stroke increases with age — it almost trebles around the age of 65 — many patients find themselves being treated under the more general umbrella of elderly care. Therefore, any nurse, from virtually any speciality, could find himself or herself involved in this area of nursing care at any time.

This article is aimed not only at nurses already working in this discipline but also at the general nurse who could be called upon to assess and care for a patient who has neurological impairment as a result of stroke.

INITIAL ASSESSMENT

The importance of the initial nursing assessment cannot be overemphasised. The purpose of this assessment is to determine the patient's state of health, mental state and lifestyle before the stroke, referred to as the pre-morbid state. Subsequent nursing care will then be three-dimensional:

- Nursing intervention, to minimise complications such as subluxation (or partial dislocation) of the shoulder, which can be the most vulnerable and physical manifestation of cerebral vascular accident
- Rehabilitation, to help the patient and family adapt to disability and altered lifestyle
- Health promotion, such as stop-smoking and dietary advice, to minimise the risk of secondary stroke.

The most important skill that a nurse can bring to bear is observation, as patients can take some time to come to terms with their condition and may not readily admit to problems. The nurse must be sensitive to such considerations as the general well-being of the patient, posture and balance when sitting, neglect by the patient of the affected side, facial droop, dribbling, swelling of the fingers on the affected side and signs of fatigue.

Much can be learnt by observing the patient at mealtimes when such problems as visual defects are most apparent. You cannot easily discern whether a patient has read a whole page of a book, but a half-eaten plate of food may be tangible evidence of a neurological defect.

Observation cannot provide all the information the nurse needs to know about the patient. Certain kinds of information, such as the amount of sensation in the hand and fingers on the affected side, can be gathered by talking to him or her. As well as indicating the extent to which the patient can understand and retain information, the process will also help to form a therapeutic relationship between nurse and patient.

The patient's condition must be quantified during or shortly after the initial assessment using a tool such as the Barthel Index, designed to measure physical function (Mahoney and Barthel, 1965). The degree to which subsequent intervention has succeeded can be determined by subsequent Barthel scores taken during treatment and before discharge.

After this initial nursing assessment, continual monitoring is maintained so that the care plan is under constant review. This process is vital for an individualised approach as stroke survivors vary so widely, both in terms of their presenting symptoms and in their responses to treatment.

Team working

Rehabilitation is a problem-solving educational process by which a disabled person achieves optimal physical, psychological and social function (Greenwood and McMillan, 1993). To achieve this, teamwork is important for maintaining continuity across all disciplines. The patient will be relearning and practising basic life skills through a process of repetition, which requires patience on the part of the staff as well as the patient. All staff will be called on to go over tasks such as washing, dressing and transferring again and again until the patient has become proficient.

Fig 5. Positioning of the patient after stroke

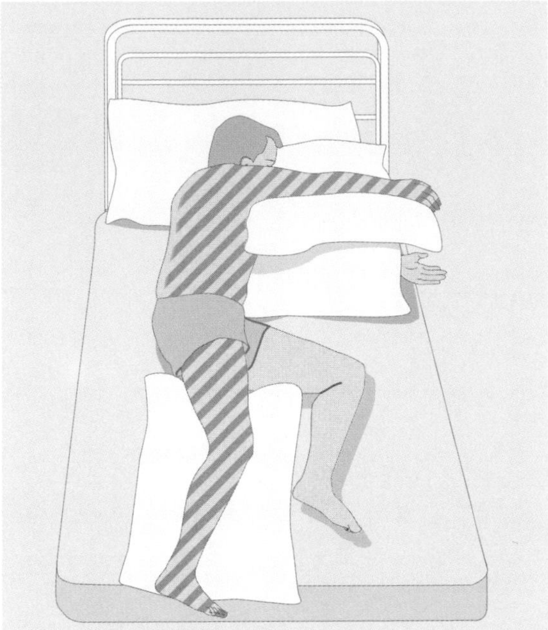

Lying on the unaffected side
The patient's head is in line with the body
The patient is fully on their side
Affected shoulder is brought forward with arm on pillow
Unaffected arm is under pillow and arms are kept parallel

Care should be taken to ensure that the patient does not over-exert himor herself on the unaffected side. The compensatory overuse of the unaffected side will increase the tone, causing spasticity on the affected side.

The patient is motivated through the setting and achieving of challenging yet realistic goals. These should be mutually agreed between the team, the patient and any relatives involved. Subsequent nursing care and therapy will then be directed towards achieving these goals. This requires carefully managed communication.

Stroke patients may spend a long time in hospital. This time needs to be structured. Patients who are involved in making decisions about how their day is spent are likely to be more positive about their treatment.

Therapists should plan their day according to a timetable which the patient is aware of. This will give the patient a feeling of autonomy and involvement in planning the day. Relatives should also be familiar with the timetable, either so that they can participate in therapy or so that visiting times can be arranged around it.

Discharge planning

Discharge planning begins immediately and is part of the initial assessment. This will entail looking at the home environment in order to determine what kinds of equipment and external assistance will be needed. If, for instance, the only toilet is upstairs or outside, the patient will need a commode. Help may be needed with washing, dressing, food preparation and housework. The kind of social care required must also be assessed, bearing in mind whether the patient is likely to remain housebound or will be able to attend a day centre or stroke club.

As part of preparation for the discharge, patients and their relatives can be encouraged gradually to relinquish their dependency on the safe hospital environment. This can be achieved through a series of short preparatory visits home, perhaps involving an overnight stay. Potential problems can then be highlighted and dealt with.

SPECIALIST NURSING INTERVENTION

It cannot be overemphasised how important correct positioning and handling of the affected limbs are in preventing such complications as contractures and painful joints (Fig 5 and 6). Normal tone, that is the slight tension within the muscle which concentrates the effect of gravity, is adversely affected following a stroke.

The nurse, together with the physiotherapist, must facilitate movements of the limbs within a pain-free range, while maintaining alignment. When placing the affected hand and arm in position, it should be done purposefully so that the patient experiences the sensation and effect of that normal movement.

Positioning the affected shoulder in sitting and lying position

A flaccid (low tone) shoulder is in permanent danger of subluxation (partial dislocation) and may become painful if poorly managed. A painful shoulder may not respond to analgesia, and the patient will be more concerned with guarding the arm and shoulder than in participating in therapy. This will have an adverse effect because everyday tasks, such as washing and dressing, will be a painful experience. Sleep may also be affected.

In sitting, place a pillow under the affected arm with the hand in front facing downwards to the patient's midline. The pillow takes the weight of the arm, thereby supporting the shoulder and holding the joint in place. The patient should be encouraged to look after the affected arm. Careful positioning also applies when lying in bed, where the shoulder needs to be supported. The patient should be encouraged to touch the affected hand, thereby promoting awareness and increasing sensation.

The patient may easily tire in the early stages of treatment. The first indication of this may be that the patient is having problems maintaining a sitting balance. This in turn will affect the patient's tone. It is good practice to build in rest periods between therapy and treatment times, gradually increasing the lengths of time sitting as patient's exercise tolerance and concentration improves.

Seating needs to be comfortable and provide a good base of support. The assessment of suitable seating falls within the scope of the physiotherapist and occupational therapist. The patient's hips, knees and ankles should be at an angle of 90 degrees when sitting.

Positioning within the ward

Stroke patients often neglect their affected side, especially if they have visual impairment, and they need to be encouraged to turn their head both ways. If possible, try to position patients with the affected side towards the ward activity to encourage awareness of that side.

ACTIVITIES OF DAILY LIVING

To a greater of lesser extent a stroke will have an impact on most or all facets of the way someone lives his or her life. Those discussed here outline the more commonly encountered experiences of people who have had a stroke.

Swallowing

Two major threats to the health and safety of the dysphagic patient are malnutrition and aspiration. Difficulty with swallowing (dysphagia) may result in difficulty with eating and an unreliable or absent swallow reflex. Eating and drinking need to be reintroduced with caution as chest infection could delay recovery or threaten survival.

A baseline weight and early referral to a dietitian is beneficial. The speech and language therapist will be able to complete an assessment of swallowing. However, a nurse may be the first to highlight problems, for example, a patient pocketing food in the mouth or a delay in swallowing. The person can be taught to check his or her mouth with the tongue if pocketing is a problem.

Fluids are more difficult to control than solids when swallowing. The speech therapist, together with a dietitian, may suggested adding a thickener to improve control. The nurse needs to be aware of the risk that a patient is silently aspirating, particularly if there are repeated chest infections or if the patient is coughing. It should be noted whether the voice sounds wet or 'gurgly' after eating or drinking and this must be reported to medical staff, as more complex assessment may be required.

If the patient is unable to swallow, he or she may require nasogastric feeding. A sudden and rapid loss of weight will be detrimental, even to an obese person. The dietitian should be involved from the outset to ensure a correct calorific regime. However, nasogastric feeding should be considered only as a short-term measure because it can be distressing, and a restless or confused patient may dislodge the tube.

The swallow assessment by the speech and language therapist should be ongoing. Long-term management might entail the insertion of a gastrostomy tube (PEG) where the patient's fluid balance and nutritional status could be more closely monitored.

Communication

The extent to which communication will be adversely affected depends on the site and side of stroke. Communication problems may be receptive, where the patient has difficulty in understanding speech, or expressive, where the patient has difficulty in speaking and in expressing him or herself. The terms aphasia and dysphasia indicate a total lack of (aphasia) or difficulty with (dysphasia) the comprehension or production of communication.

However, apparently profound problems can sometimes be alleviated by such simple measures as checking that hearing aids are working properly and that dentures are properly fitted. Enlisting the expertise of the speech and language therapist again ensures that a fuller assessment is carried out and the appropriate treatment approach prescribed. Nursing staff can remind patients to practise exercises learnt in therapy sessions.

Communication cards and boards should be issued with caution. If the patient is unable to understand how to use them this will only add to the frustration.

Stroke patients frequently confuse their yes and no responses. Closed questions requiring such responses should be avoided where possible. When communicating, speak slowly, using short phrases and simple language but without descending into baby talk. The nurse must be sure that he or she has the patient's attention before speaking and establish eye contact if possible.

The most important things a nurse can give stroke patients are time and patience, while promoting an environment as free from distraction as possible.

Washing and dressing assessment

The everyday tasks of washing and dressing are complex sequences of activities which have to be learnt. Because they have many components, they are good basic assessments of overall function. The nurse will probably be the first to note any difficulties in this area, whereupon the occupational therapist may decide to proceed with a more complex assessment, such as the Rivermead Perceptual Test, a battery of tests covering eight categories, including sequencing, body image and inattention (Friedman and Leong, 1992)

Elimination

Continence is often used as an indicator of recovery after a stroke. It is common for the patient to have continence problems in the first 24 hours, especially if the overall condition is poor. Patients may need to be catheterised in the early stages, although this can create certain problems, including risk of infection. The catheter should be removed as soon as possible as part of the rehabilitation process.

Diminished sensation in the bowel following a stroke may lead to constipation. This can increase spasticity. Loss of sensation may also result in overflow diarrhoea which, as well as demoralising the patient, limits participation in rehabilitation sessions.

The nurse has a role in ensuring that the patient is given the opportunity to use the toilet at times established by their pre-morbid routine and by monitoring frequency of movements.

HEALTH PROMOTION

To prevent recurrence potential risk factors should be identified and managed after discharge. The nurse has an educative role in encouraging the patients to comply with continuing treatment and to minimise risk factors.

The nurse should work with the pharmacist to ensure that patient and carer understand the purpose of medication and potential complications that may arise. The most likely forms of drug therapy are antihypertensives and, where the stroke was caused by a thrombus rather than haemorrhage, anticoagulants such as aspirin.

The nurse should also enlist the help of the dietitian in encouraging the patient to reduce fat and cholesterol intake. This must be within realistic limits. For the overweight person, the benefits of weight loss should be emphasised. Patients should also be encouraged to give up smoking or at least cut down. Patient and carer need to understand this, but preaching or adopting a judgemental attitude is likely to be counter-productive.

THINKING POINTS

- **How is the care of a patient who has had a stroke organised and could it be arranged more effectively?**
- **How do you regard people who have had strokes?**

PART THREE

Professional issues

Despite all the efforts of recent years resulting in stroke treatment becoming recognised as a specialty, the effect of different types of treatment remains unclear (Wolfe et al, 1995). In this final section, we shall look at a selection of contentious areas, including the attitude of non-specialist staff and how this affects management of stroke patients.

HOSPITAL VERSUS HOME TREATMENT

In the UK stroke usually results in hospitalisation, with around 12% of all medical bed days and 25% of bed days in elderly care being accounted for by stroke patients.

However, it has been argued that many patients might

not be admitted on medical grounds, whatever it may say in their notes, but 'rather, the hospital is used as a form of rapid-access sanctuary' (Young, 1994). This is seen as a short-term approach, which concentrates on dealing with disability at the expense of tackling handicap or the way in which a disability affects the individual's ability to carry out activities of living.

In the hospital setting, the argument goes, the individual is living in an artificial environment, which may be very different from his or her home; for example, the average ward or unit is a lot bigger and less cluttered than most people's living area, and few patients will have nurses in earshot for 24 hours a day on returning home. This affects the way rehabilitation is planned, with care focusing on a standardised repertoire of abilities, achievement of which is counted as 'success'. On discharge, the person may face having to adapt that repertoire to very different circumstances.

In the 1970s, a researcher looked at the way people with one of a range of newly diagnosed disabilities, which included stroke, managed after discharge from hospital and described the lifestyle changes that each had to make, both soon after arriving home and over the longer term, a process which she described as like undertaking 'a career in disability' (Blaxter, 1980).

More recently, Young has argued that little has changed since then, believing that the hospital-based view of discharge as being the end of rehabilitation has forced patients into 'careers in stroke' (Young, 1994). Emphasis put on physical recovery leads to neglect of 'the competing needs of education, psychological support and enhancing social opportunities for patients and families'. Young cites Holbrook's model of stroke recovery, in which the victim passes through the stage of crisis, through treatment and realisation and finally attains adjustment, saying that in hospital many patients never get beyond treatment stage (Holbrook, 1982).

The answer, proposed by more than one expert, has been the setting up of community-based stroke services once their effectiveness had been proven in large-scale research studies. Such services would differ from those seen as the norm now, chiefly in that the individual's home would be central to setting goals, rather than the physiotherapist's gym or occupational therapist's treatment room.

There is little doubt that in the UK there is need for better-coordinated rehabilitation services, but the differences between all the professionals concerned militates against this (Lincoln, 1994). It might also mean that there has to be a complete reversal in the way priorities are set: at the moment in many settings, patients with the least chance of recovery often receive the highest level of input, while those who are best set for greater recovery, because their disabilities are less, receive a much lower input. In a truly coordinated stroke service, where patients would be treated along the lines of critical pathways, some very difficult decisions might have to be made. And the question of finances cannot be ducked: 'emphasis will be on cost control, not on the provision of services to the community' (Millard and Higgs, 1989).

THROMBOLYTIC TREATMENT

The success of thrombolytic therapy in the treatment of myocardial infarction has led many researchers to believe

Fig 6. Repositioning the patient who has had a stroke

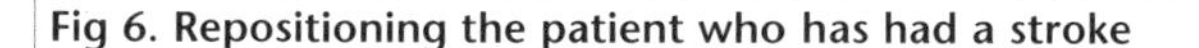

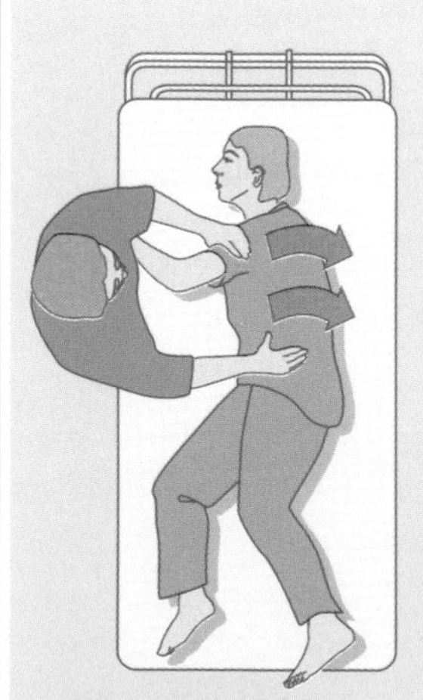

1. Remove all the pillows. Roll the patient's hip backwards so the patient rolls onto his or her back

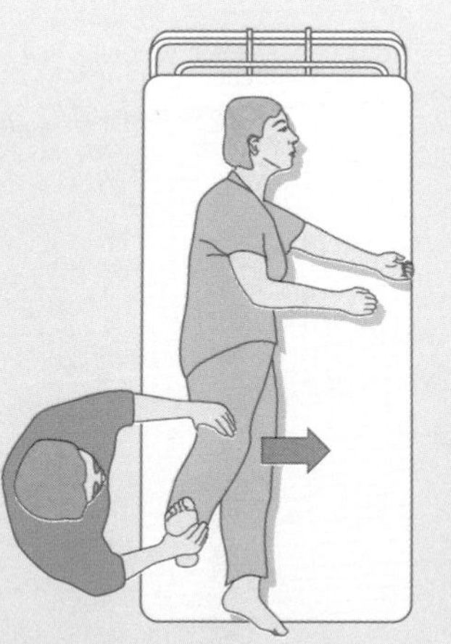

2. Turn the head to the side. Cross his or her arm over the body so that they are both on the same side. Push the hip and knee. Push the knee across the other leg

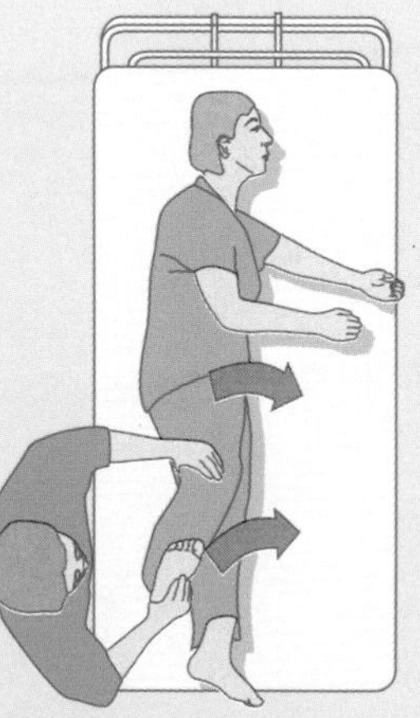

3. Lift the patient's foot across the other leg. Roll the hip forwards

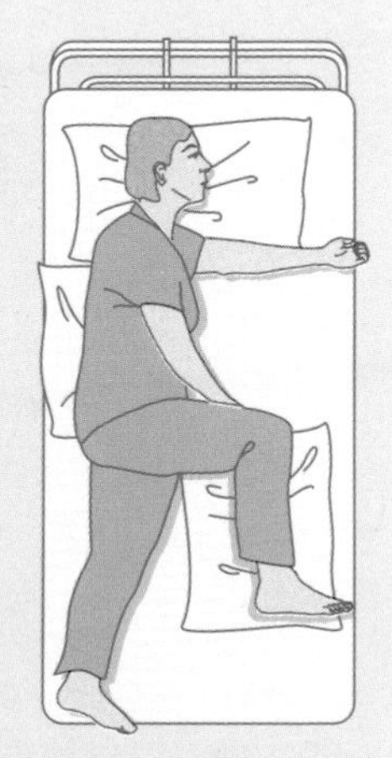

4. Reposition the patient using pillows

than an effective treatment for stroke may be within reach. However, stroke may be worsened by the use of such agents, and research has concentrated on weighing advantages against disadvantages.

One set of researchers, the MAST (Multi-centre Acute Stroke Trial) Group, has been looking at a number of treatment options, and the MAST-I group, based in Italy, conducted a trial of streptokinase and aspirin at centres in Italy, Portugal and the UK (MAST-1, 1995). This ran from May 1991 to February 1995, and, of the more than 14000 patients eligible for entry into the trial, a randomly selected 5% sample of 622 patients made up the study population.

Eligibility criteria included patients' admission to hospital within six hours after sudden onset of a stroke, with computerised tomographic (CT) scanning being performed.

Subjects were randomly assigned to one of four groups, in which they would receive either streptokinase intravenously; aspirin for 10 days; both drugs; or neither. All were closely observed for 10 days, and a second CT scan was conducted on day five or if another stroke occurred. If a patient died, details were sent to the research coordinators; in the case of survivors a telephone interview was conducted six months after discharge and their degree of recovery was assessed.

Analysis of the results showed that patients given streptokinase, either alone or with aspirin, had a higher chance of dying in the first 10 days after stroke; in the control group there was a 13% chance of fatality, but for those receiving streptokinase alone it was 19%. If both drugs were given, the mortality rate was 34%, a statistically significant figure.

But, after six months, members of the streptokinase groups were less likely to have died and had a lesser degree of disability. This may have been due, in part, to the fact that deaths in the early stages were higher, but the researchers believed that their finding of an absolute risk reduction of 50–70 deaths per 1000 patients treated, extrapolated from all the data, showed a significant benefit, pointing out that, for stroke patients and their families, severe disability might well equate with death.

Until further data are available, the MAST researchers do not recommend routine use of thrombolytic therapy in acute treatment of stroke.

This study demonstrates a particular problem in stroke treatment: if a therapy of any kind reduces the chance of future disability, but increased the possibility of death within a defined period, should it be given at all? Where do the cut-off points, if any, lie?

NURSES' ATTITUDES TO STROKE PATIENTS

Jane Williams, a ward manager in rehabilitation with a special interest in stroke, has highlighted a major problem for nurses in the specialty. 'I believe that sometimes nurses are their own worst enemies. Many of our colleagues still adopt a superior attitude to geriatric nurses. "Couldn't you get a job elsewhere?" is a common remark.' (Williams, 1993)

Gibbon looked at the attitudes towards stroke patients in general medical wards (Gibbon, 1991). He cites Stockwell's classic paper on the 'unpopular patient' (Stockwell, 1972), noting that stroke patients are often seen as being 'uncooperative, difficult to talk to, unlikely to progress' and also mentions Hamrin's finding that attitudes towards this group can be improved by education of staff (Hamrin, 1982).

Gibbon replicated the first part of Hamrin's US study, sending a five-point Likert scale questionnaire to 84 members of staff in the medical wards of a teaching hospital (53 registered nurses, 19 enrolled nurses and 12 nursing auxiliaries). After follow-up, 76 (90.5%) were completed and returned.

Analysis showed that most staff, irrespective of grade, had attitudes towards stroke patients that were not particularly negative or positive. However, the more motivated registered nurses felt more strongly that better rehabilitation would be possible with higher staffing levels and expressed a concern that more input into work with stroke patients could lead to other groups being neglected. The auxiliaries laid more stress on the uncooperative nature of stroke patients.

Gibbon concludes that there is still a lot of work to be done in clarifying what is meant by the idea of nurses as rehabilitators, noting that they would probably become more motivated in this area if they knew more about it.

It has not proved possible to find any data on this, but it seems reasonable to assume that many patients who receive treatment in specialised stroke units do not always arrive there within 48 hours of the stroke. This means that they are awaiting transfer from wards in which, if they are not viewed positively, the best that can be hoped for is ambivalence — hardly a good start in rehabilitation.

More research remains to be done in this area, which appears to have many similarities to the way accident victims have been treated — what happened on site was considered unimportant, because 'real' treatment began as soon as they reached hospital. Now there is the concept of the 'golden hour', in which the initial stages after injury are seen as all-important: perhaps there needs to be a similar shift in attitudes towards the treatment of stroke patients.

PREVENTING STROKE

The *Our Healthier Nation* document set national targets for the reduction of risk factors in stroke. The medical consensus is that, in principle, stroke is preventable. This is based on three sets of data (Marmot and Poulter, 1993).

- Time trends: death rates have fallen greatly in recent decades in Western industrialised countries and Japan but have risen in some Eastern European countries. The factor or factors involved have not been identified

- National differences in stroke mortality are not fixed; for example, the descendants of migrants tend to be affected to the same degree as the indigenous population with time
- The causes of stroke identified in recent years are often avoidable and their effects reversible; it has been suggested that 50% of all cerebrovascular deaths in patients under 70 years might be preventable by application of existing knowledge.

Risk factors identified to date can be broadly grouped under the following headings:

- Fixed biological: for example, age and sex
- Malleable biological: including blood pressure, blood glucose concentration, serum cholesterol level
- Individual behavioural: for example, smoking, diet, alcohol use
- Social/ethnic
- Environmental factors.

These are not discrete groups; for example, an individual's social class may make him or her more likely to be a smoker, which in turn affects blood pressure; that in itself might be determined by genetic factors, possibly affected by racial characteristics.

Yet the Department of Health apparently believes that its targets are attainable. A paper which appeared the year before Health of the Nation suggested some 'practical priorities' (Marmot, 1993). These included a mean reduction of 5mmHg in blood pressure for the whole population, by reducing sodium intake, reducing body mass indices and getting heavy drinkers to cut down their intake of alcohol; and closer monitoring of blood pressure in primary care, with the aim of increasing the proportion of people with hypertension whose condition is under control

For the health care worker, all sorts of problems are raised by the ideal of health promotion, and it is particularly noticeable in the field of stroke treatment. The risk factors are not cut and dried; for example, no one really understands the link between cholesterol levels and stroke, although the health pages of many popular publications do not give any impression of uncertainty — so advice given to patients on lifestyle changes, based on available knowledge, can sound rather vague. This may lead to accusations of 'health fascism' a term which carries overtones of unjustified infringement of the individual's rights.

It may be easy to explain to an obese person why reducing their weight will help with their rehabilitation and how the chance of another stroke will be reduced. But how can the dangers inherent in smoking be easily explained, especially if the person does not want to listen? And how does one counter claims that the person has only limited years left to live, so why give up a pleasurable activity?

It is not simply a matter of telling people what to do: it is about working in partnership, building up trust and telling the truth in a way that can not only be understood but is seen as not being selective with the facts.

As the specialty grows there will be an ever-expanding number of other difficult areas. But if the challenges did not exist, nursing stroke patients would not be anywhere near as rewarding as it is.

REFERENCES

Andrews, K. (1987) *Rehabilitation of the Older Adult*. London: Edward Arnold.
Blaxter, M. (1980) *Meaning of Disability*. London: Heinemann.
Booth, B. (1994) The knowledge nurses need to educate patients about stroke. *Nursing Times*; 90: 15, 32–33.
Friedman, P.J., Leong, L. (1992) The Perceptive Assessment Battery in acute stroke. *British Journal of Occupational Therapy*; 55: 6, 233–237.
Gibbon, B. (1991) A reassessment of nurses' attitudes towards stroke patients in general medical wards. *Journal of Advanced Nursing*; 16: 1336–1342.
Greenwood, R.J., McMillan, T.M. (1993) Models of rehabilitation programmes for the brain-injured adult: Part 1. *Clinical Rehabilitation*; 7: 3, 248—255.
Hamrin, E. (1982) Attitudes of nurses staffing general medical wards towards activation of stroke patients. *Journal of Advanced Nursing*; 7: 33–42.
Hedley, R. (1994) *Voices for Stroke*. London: Stroke Association.
Holbrook, M. (1982) Stroke and emotional outcome. *Journal of the Royal College of Physicians of London*; 16: 100–104.
King, P. (1990) *Living with Stroke*. Manchester: Manchester University Press.
Lincoln, N.B. (1994) Is stroke better managed in the community? *British Medical Journal*; 309: 1357–1358.
Mahoney, R.I., Barthel, D.W. (1965) Barthel Index. Brisbane: University of Queensland.
Marmot, M.G., Poulter, N.R. (1992) Primary prevention of stroke. *Lancet*; 339: 344–347.
MAST-I (1995) Randomised controlled trial of streptokinase, aspirin, and a combination of both in the treatment of acute ischaemic stroke. *Lancet*; 346: 1509–1514.
Millard, P., Higgs, P. (1989) The future and care of the elderly. *Care of the Elderly*; 1: 6, 284–285.
Sacks, O. (1986) *The Man Who Mistook His Wife for a Hat*. London: Picador.
Stockwell, F. (1972) *The Unpopular Patient*. London: RCN.
Swaffield, L. (1990) *Stroke: The Complete Guide to Recovery and Rehabilitation*. Wellingborough: Thorsons.
Williams, J. (1993) Rehabilitation challenge. *Nursing Times*; 89: 66–70.
Wolfe, C.D.A. et al (1995) Stroke care in Europe. *Journal of the Royal Society of Health*; 115: 3, 143–147.
World Health Organization (1971) *Cerebrovascular Diseases: Prevention, Treatment and Rehabilitation*. Geneva: WHO.
Young, J. (1994) Is stroke better managed in the community? *British Medical Journal*; 309: 1356–1357.

Useful address

Stroke Association
Stroke House
Whitecross Street
London EC1Y 8JJ
Tel: 0171 566 0300

Stroke

Assessment

When you have read the unit and completed any further reading, you can use the questions below to test your understanding of the topic. Answers can be found on the next page.

1. In the league table of fatal diseases in the Western world, stroke comes:

- [ ] 1 First
- [ ] 2 Second
- [ ] 3 Third
- [ ] 4 Fourth

2. The *Our Healthier Nation* initiative set a target of reducing the incidence of stroke by a minimum of:

- [ ] 1 10%
- [ ] 2 25%
- [ ] 3 40%
- [ ] 4 55%

3. The area of the brain connected with speech is called:

- [ ] 1 Wernicke's area
- [ ] 2 Broca's area
- [ ] 3 Sack's area
- [ ] 4 Spooner's area

4. Homonymous heminopia affects:

- [ ] 1 Half of the visual field in each eye
- [ ] 2 Half of the visual field of the eye on the affected side
- [ ] 3 All of the visual field on the affected side and half of the visual field on the unaffected side
- [ ] 4 One eye only

5. The number of people who are estimated to experience a stroke every year in the UK is:

- [ ] 1 85 000
- [ ] 2 110 000
- [ ] 3 135 000
- [ ] 4 160 000

6. Mortality from stroke is:

- [ ] 1 Going up in all parts of the world
- [ ] 2 Is falling in the Western world because of improved health promotion
- [ ] 3 Is impossible to improve
- [ ] 4 Is falling in Western countries but rising in Eastern Europe

7. By definition, a transient ischaemic attack lasts:

- [ ] 1 Less than six hours
- [ ] 2 More than six but less than 12 hours
- [ ] 3 Less than 24 hours
- [ ] 4 More than 24 hours but less than 48

8. The most common cause of stroke is:

- [ ] 1 Thrombosis
- [ ] 2 Embolus
- [ ] 3 Haemorrhage
- [ ] 4 Stress

9. Not recognising a part of the body as one's own is known as:

- [ ] 1 Apraxia
- [ ] 2 Ataxia
- [ ] 3 Anosmia
- [ ] 4 Anosognosia

10. A stroke affecting the posterior cerebral artery is likely to result in:

- [ ] 1 Upper limb weakness
- [ ] 2 Lower limb weakness
- [ ] 3 Visual loss
- [ ] 4 Dysphagia

11. The term spasticity can be defined as:

- [ ] 1 A tendency to spasm
- [ ] 2 Lowered muscle tone
- [ ] 3 Excessive muscle flexion
- [ ] 4 Loss of coordination

12. The cardiac condition most closely associated with stroke aetiology is:

- [ ] 1 Ventricular fibrillation
- [ ] 2 Atrial fibrillation
- [ ] 3 Myocardial infarction
- [ ] 4 Heart block

13 Neuroplasticity is a process in which:

- 1 Undamaged areas of the brain take over the work of damaged areas
- 2 New nerve tissues develop
- 3 Nerve fibres may be bent without breaking
- 4 Unmyelinated nerves develop a myelin sheath

14 When a stroke is evolving, neurological deficits usually worsen for:

- 1 Up to 24 hours
- 2 Between 24 and 48 hours
- 3 Between 48 and 72 hours
- 4 Without time limit

15 In dysarthria, as opposed to dysphasia, the problem:

- 1 Lies in the cortex
- 2 Stems from inability to understand spoken words
- 3 Is mechanical
- 4 Affects hearing and speech

ANSWERS

Stroke

1: In the league table of fatal diseases in the Western world, stroke comes:
3) Third

2: The *Our Healthier Nation* initiative set a target of reducing the incidence of stroke by a minimum of:
3) 40%

3: The area of the brain connected with speech is called:
2) Broca's area

4: Homonymous heminopia affects:
1) Half of the visual field in each eye

5: The number of people who are estimated to experience a stroke very year in the UK is:
2) 110 000

6: Mortality from stroke is:
4)Is falling in Western countries but rising in Eastern Europe

7: By definition, a transient ischaemic attack lasts:
3) Less than 24 hours

8: The most common cause of stroke is:
1) Thrombosis

9: Not recognising a part of the body as one's own is known as:
1) Apraxia

10: A stroke affecting the posterior cerebral artery is likely to result in:
3) Visual loss

11:The term spasticity can be defined as:
3) Excessive muscle flexion

12: The cardiac condition most closely associated with stroke aetiology is:
3) Myocardial infarction

13: Neuroplasticity is a process in which:
1) Undamaged areas of the brain take over the work of damaged areas

14: When a stroke is evolving, neurological deficits usually worsen for:
4) Without time limit

15: In dysarthria, as opposed to dysphasia, the problem:
3) Is mechanical

Fractured neck of femur

Knowledge for practice

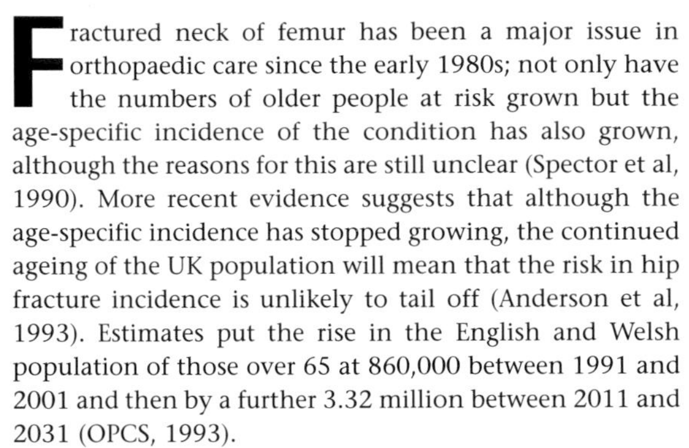

Fractured neck of femur has been a major issue in orthopaedic care since the early 1980s; not only have the numbers of older people at risk grown but the age-specific incidence of the condition has also grown, although the reasons for this are still unclear (Spector et al, 1990). More recent evidence suggests that although the age-specific incidence has stopped growing, the continued ageing of the UK population will mean that the risk in hip fracture incidence is unlikely to tail off (Anderson et al, 1993). Estimates put the rise in the English and Welsh population of those over 65 at 860,000 between 1991 and 2001 and then by a further 3.32 million between 2011 and 2031 (OPCS, 1993).

Fractured neck of femur will place an increasing strain on orthopaedic and geriatric services, especially as the ageing population is not only likely to be more prone to fractures but will require more intensive care after the fracture because of their increased frailty.

By the time they are 90, it has been estimated that one in three women and one in six men will have had a fractured neck of femur. The mortality for hip fractures is relatively high and it is estimated that the annual mortality in the UK is 7,500 or 15% of the total having a fracture. The most common underlying pathology is loss of bone density — osteoporosis. Factors increasing the risk of hip fracture are showing in Table 1.

ANATOMY OF THE HIP

The femur forms part of the appendicular skeleton and is the longest and strongest bone in the body. As the upper end is set at an angle of about 120° to the rest of the bone, and since the weight of the entire body is borne by the two femora, fracture of the bone close to the upper end, or the neck, is most common.

At its upper end, the femur fits into the acetabulum, the cup-shaped socket on the pelvis, forming the hip joint. At its lower end the femur meets the tibia and patella in the knee joint.

The neck of the femur is a pyramidal-shaped section of bone, connecting the shaft of the femur at the greater and lesser trochanters, the name given to the two bony promi-

Fig 1. A: regions where hip fractures may occur: the head and neck of the femur and the trochanteric regions. B: intracapsular fracture across the neck

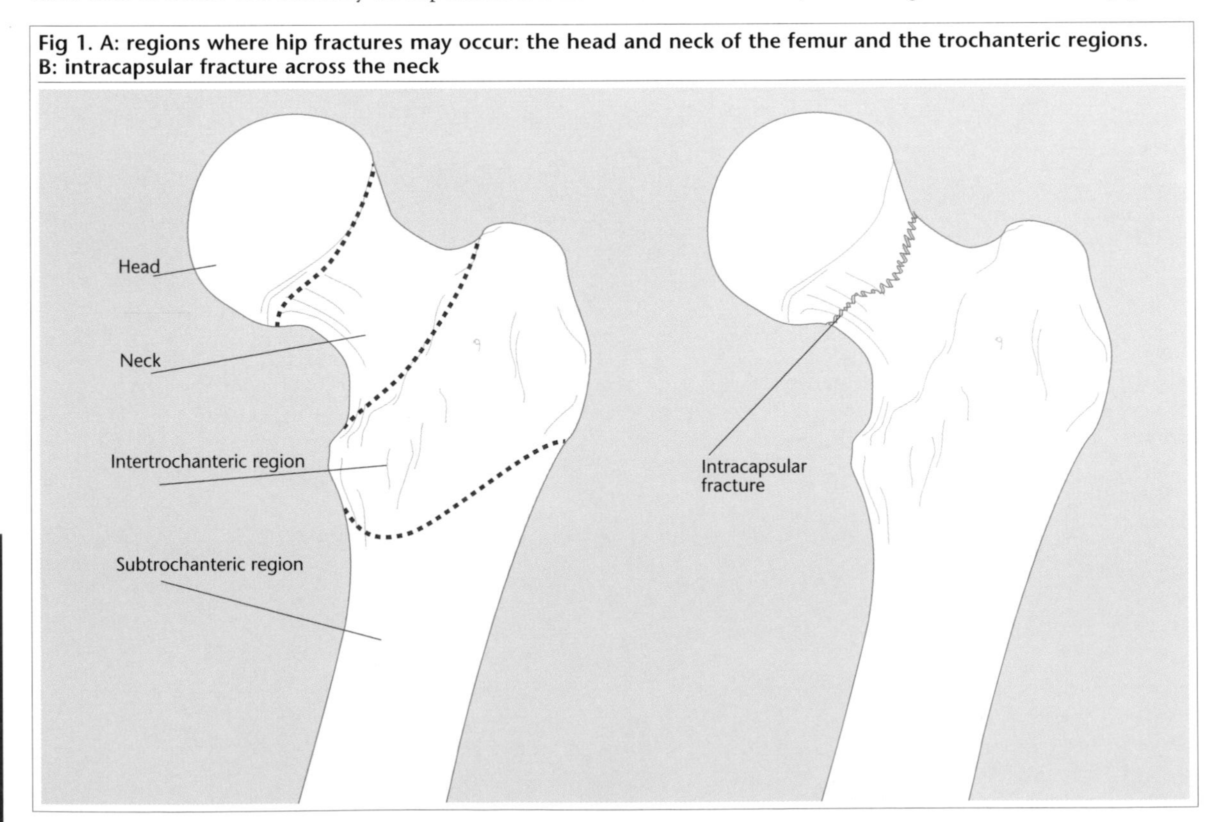

Table. 1 Factors increasing the risk of hip fracture

● Osteoporosis	● Smoking
● Low body weight	● High protein, alcohol or caffeine consumption
● Age	● Bone cancer
● Low activity involving weight-bearing	● Confusion
● Low dietary calcium and vitamin D	● Prolonged bed rest

nences at the upper end of the thigh bone. The greater trochanter can be felt on the outer side of the thigh while the lesser trochanter is a small prominence on the inner side of the bone.

The articular capsule of the hip joint is made of dense, fibrous tissue, lined with synovial membrane and articular cartilage. The capsule extends from the acetabulum to the intertrochanteric line anteriorally. Posteriorally it covers two-thirds of the neck. The position of the fracture in relation to the capsule is used to classify different types of hip fracture.

CLINICAL FEATURES AND TYPES OF FRACTURE

Fractures of the femoral neck can happen even with no injury at all: the bones of some people become so brittle that a fracture can occur as they lift themselves out of a chair. It has been calculated that four-fifths of femoral neck fractures in England and Wales are at least partially attributable to the reduction in bone mass that occurs with age.

Intracapsular fractures (Fig 1)

These fractures will allow the shaft of the femur to move independently of the hip joint. Therefore on examination the affected limb will be short but also the iliopsoas muscle and gravity will rotate the bone externally instead of internally.

Fractures which occur within the articular capsule are termed intracapsular. These include:

- Subcapital fractures — distal to the articular margin of the head of the femur
- Transcervical fractures — through the neck
- Basal fractures — at the base of the neck.

Intracapsular fractures result from a high transcervical fracture and may interrupt the blood supply to the femoral head, which is supplied via the capsule, the medullary cavity and from the ligamentum teres. Such a fracture can result in the blood supply to the femoral head being cut off completely.

This can lead to aseptic necrosis, non-union or both and because the fracture line is actually inside the capsule, blood can become trapped within it. This raises the intracapsular pressure, causing more damage to the femoral head, although no bruising is visible because blood is not able to reach the subcutaneous tissue.

Another problem is caused by the fact that this type of fracture leaves the femoral head extremely mobile in the capsule. This makes accurate reduction almost impossible and the posterior cortex may be crushed. These problems are why intracapsular fractures are much more likely to have high complication rates.

Extracapsular fractures

Extracapsular fractures occur across the trochanteric region of the femur. They tend to be less difficult than intracapsular fractures because the blood supply is not as significantly interrupted.

The surface area of the break is greater and gives a better chance of union as well as consisting of good cancellous bone — the term applied to loose bony tissue at the end of all long bones. Despite this, non-union and necrosis can occur.

Undisplaced and impacted fractures of the neck of femur

These can be a problem because they can remain undiagnosed. As the bones are packed tightly together, the break can appear stable. The patient may even be able to bear weight on the leg.

Although many patients will do very well without treatment, in some the fracture can become displaced days or even weeks after the injury.

An impacted fracture must be carefully observed to make sure it remains stable. The neck should be protected until union.

TREATMENT OPTIONS

Fractures can be treated by internal fixation or prosthetic replacement. The choice of procedure depends largely on the age of the patient and how fit he or she is. Other major factors include the type of fracture (see above) and the degree to which the fracture is displaced.

Internal fixation

Most hip fractures are repaired by a procedure termed open reduction internal fixation or ORIF. It involves the surgeon making an incision and then realigning the fracture, which is then secured with pins, nails, screws or plates. This process is also referred to as compression with dynamic screw and plate. Image intensification is used to guide the surgeon.

Open reduction internal fixation is most suitable for fractures in the intertrochanteric or subtrochanteric regions. Internal fixation is most suitable for basal fractures where the largest fractures take place.

After internal fixation, the limb must be protected from full weight-bearing; this may be particularly difficult in older patients.

If the procedure is successful it can result in an almost perfect hip. But the surgery can be complicated by aseptic necrosis or mal-union.

In these cases a prosthesis will be required, involved a

second operation. Another complication is that the head may collapse on to the pins and so damage the acetabulum.

Prosthetic replacement

If blood supply to the femoral head is disrupted, aseptic necrosis to the head is likely. In these cases, or if there is serious displacement, a prosthetic replacement is more likely. Immediate replacement of the head avoids the complication of mal-union and allows immediate full weight-bearing. If damage or arthritis is found in the acetabulum the surgeon may also replace the socket cup.

If either the femoral head or the acetabulum is replaced, the procedure is called a hemi-arthroplasty. If both are replaced it is termed a total arthroplasty.

It is a feature of all prosthetic replacements that, if successful, the results are better than other techniques. But if unsuccessful they are invariably worse (Pellino, 1994).

OUTCOME AND COMPLICATIONS

More than 95% of patients have surgery to repair their fracture (Todd et al, 1995). Most patients do very well, but in England and Wales in 1990, fractured neck of femur was responsible for 1,155 deaths, with an additional 416 deaths due to other unspecified similar fractures (OPCS, 1993). Other adverse events, such as infection, thrombo-embolism in the leg and pressure sores cause many problems.

After their internal fixation or prosthetic replacement the patient will have a drain in place for at least two days and during that time will probably be given antibiotics intravenously to reduce infection.

The issue of prophylaxis against thrombo-embolism in hospital patients in general has been a controversial one. But evidence has accrued over the past decade that such prophylaxis is life-saving in preventing non-fatal symptomatic thrombo-embolism requiring investigation and treatment (THRIFT, 1992). For patients with hip fractures, prophylaxis is recommended with either warfarin or dextran 70. Each of these methods prevents 40 to 50% of deep vein thrombi and reduces the risk of pulmonary embolism.

In patients with heart disease, warfarin may be preferred because dextran may increase the risk of fluid overload in older patients.

Fixed low-dose heparin is the usual recommended prophylaxis for prevention of deep-vein thrombosis but its use has not been shown to be useful in patients with fractured neck of femur. However, there have been encouraging trials of low molecular weight heparins for these patients.

REDUCING THE STRAIN ON THE NHS

Hip fractures are placing an increasing economic strain on the NHS. This could be countered by an increase in the efficacy of surgical and rehabilitative techniques. Average pre-convalescent length of stay has already been significantly reduced from 37.3 days in 1979 to 29.7 days in 1985 (Department of Health, 1989).

If further cost savings are to be made, it is estimated that all patients would have to be discharged from all types of hospital care within 19 days of admission (Hollingworth et al, 1995). The reduction in length of stay achieved between 1979 and 1985 is unlikely to be sustainable.

One review of interventions concluded that regular weight-bearing exercise and the cessation of smoking could have a major impact on hip fracture incidence by increasing bone mass at the younger age or reducing loss of bone mass (Law et al, 1991). Regular exercise would reduce the risk of hip fracture by at least half which could result in a drop of 20,000 cases of hip fracture every year in the UK. Women who stop smoking before the menopause reduce their risk of a fracture by around a quarter.

The value of hormone replacement therapy (HRT) in reducing the risk of fracture has been controversial. Post-menopausal oestrogen replacement reduces the risk by almost half but the protection lasts no longer than a few years after stopping treatment. Calcium supplementation is not thought to be justified as the likely benefit is too small.

Screening the population to identify those at most risk, that is, by measuring bone mineral density, has not yet been shown to be cost-effective.

The role of drugs in treating osteoporosis has again been controversial. Many studies have shown increases in bone mass with treatments such as oestrogen (Lufuin et al, 1992), calcitonin (Overgaard et al, 1992), calcitriol (Tilyard et al, 1992), sodium fluoride (Pak et al, 1995) and bisphosphonates (Storm et al, 1990). But it was only recently that any treatment, in this case, alendronate, has been shown to reduce the risk of hip fracture (Black et al, 1997). That study showed that in women with a previous fracture and low bone mass, treatment with alendronate reduced the risk of fracture in the spine and wrist as well as the hip.

Trying to prevent falls by modifying the environment of patients will be discussed in part two, but at least one study has shown that trying to prove the benefit of these changes is not straightforward (Gibson et al, 1987).

CONCLUSION

Finding solutions to the challenge of the increasing number of hip fractures is becoming ever more urgent. Either extra hospital beds or major initiatives will be needed to prevent fracture, improve treatment and provide for community care. These aspects and the role of the nurse within them will be discussed in parts two and three.

THINKING POINT

- **Apart from age, what factors contribute to the increased incidence of fractured neck of femur?**

The role of the nurse

Hip fracture poses a significant and growing challenge to the health and social services, with 57,000 people sustaining fractures each year at an estimated cost for hospital treatment of £250 million.

Unless treatment patterns change or the incidence falls, the same study has estimated the cost in 2011 as being £360 million (at 1991 prices), with 68,894 cases needing 539,000 extra hospital days per year. That figure would rise to 96,000 cases in 2031, costing £507 million to treat, and call for over 1.6 million extra bed days per year (Hollingworth et al, 1995).

If the NHS is to be able to cope with this increase it is essential that best practice is adopted as widely as possible. Surgical techniques have improved over the past decade and the majority of fractures can now be treated surgically, with most patients being able to walk within a day of surgery and, with planned rehabilitation and home support, be able to return home in some instances within two weeks of sustaining the fracture.

But according to an Audit Commission report (1995), if patients are to be discharged as soon as possible, with adequate community care, services must be led by a multidisciplinary team.

Both the Audit Commission report and one from the Royal College of Physicians agree that in many cases it should be the nurse who acts as coordinator. A patient-centred approach is regarded as essential, and both reports emphasise that realistic goals must be set for patients and that lines of communication between team members must be clear so that patients receive consistent advice.

CARE FOLLOWING ADMISSION

Most patients are admitted through the accident and emergency department (A&E), and are then transferred to an orthopaedic ward for surgery. While they are in the orthopaedic ward, treatment for any medical conditions will also be initiated.

Following surgery, patients will take part in a rehabilitation programme from nurses and therapy staff, either in the acute ward or in a unit especially designed for elderly care services.

Most patients will return to their own home. Others will move into sheltered housing or into residential care.

Table 2. Process of care for patients with fractured neck of femur

Admission via A&E
Surgery and treatment
Acute ward care and assessment
Rehabilitation
Discharge to own home, sheltered accommodation or residential care

ACCIDENT AND EMERGENCY

Once a patient is admitted to A&E, the A&E team's priorities are, first, to confirm the diagnosis and then to assess medical, nursing and social needs. If surgery is necessary it should be undertaken as soon as possible (Table 2).

It is recommended by the Royal Society of Physicians (1989) report that patients should not spend more than one hour in A&E. The recommendation is based on the fact that many of these patients may already have been lying for some time, undiscovered, in their home after falling and may be dehydrated and confused when admitted.

Furthermore, pressure sores can start to develop in these patients if they are lying undisturbed on a hard surface for even 30 minutes (if they were not already present on their admission).

It is difficult for pressure area care to be carried out adequately in A&E because of the staff's high workload, although A&E nurses recognise its importance.

The Audit Commission (1995) noted that only one hospital of the nine in its survey was able to X-ray patients on a soft surface.

The Commission also noted that, in principle, A&E staff agree that patients should not have to wait for more than an hour before surgery but stated that waiting for a doctor, waiting for an X-ray and then for an assessment, frequently meant delays of more than an hour. A&E departments vary in the provision they make for older patients; only a minority have a nurse specifically trained in the care of older people (Audit Commission, 1995).

SURGERY AND TREATMENT

There is a direct link between delayed operations and increased mortality and morbidity (Todd, 1995) and RCP guidelines recommend that operations should be carried out within 24 hours (RCP, 1989).

There is still a great deal of variation in how long patients wait and it is recognised that in some instances it may be better for a patient to wait more than 24 hours if, for example, it means that a more experienced surgeon will be available.

Preoperative care

The problems caused by delay can be exacerbated by denying patients food and water before surgery. Research has shown that a four-hour period is usually sufficient, but that in some units patients on a morning list are starved from midnight and those on an afternoon list from 6am (Audit Commission, 1995). However, water and food should be denied for no more than four to six hours.

This does not, of course, apply to patients who are to be given nil orally for other reasons, and the nurse should help to reduce anxiety and confusion by explaining why a patient should not eat or drink. Intravenous fluids should be given if food and drink are withheld for longer than eight hours. Good liaison between surgeon, theatre and ward staff should mean that delays can be foreseen so that appropriate action can be taken.

Details of the types of fractured neck of femur and their

Table 3. Key information that should be obtained during an assessment

Pressure sore risk

A validated risk assessment tool should be used to highlight the risk factors:

- Dehydration
- Body weight
- Debilitating disorders
- Poor nutrition
- Trauma and surgery
- Reduced mobility
- Pain
- Discoloured or broken skin
- Poorly managed continence

Hydration and nutrition

- Consider nutritional risk factors — nutritional status can be affected by physical, economic and social constraints.

Pain

- Use a pain assessment tool to provide an objective measure of pain
- Determine whether patient also has chronic pain from other conditions

Continence

Possible causes of incontinence include:

- Constipation
- Urinary infection
- Pelvic floor damage
- Neurological disease

Each will require a different plan of care.

Co-existing medical problems

- Check medical history — respiratory and cardiac disorders may highlight that particular attention should be paid to type of anaesthesia given
- Check current medication
- Involve patients and carers
- Involve GP and district nurses, if appropriate.

Mental state

- Assess carefully cause of confusion — this may not necessarily be dementia but may be a result of pain or dehydration
- Cognitive function can be assessed by simple tools:
  - the geriatric depression score
  - the mini mental state examination
- Lifestyle and past history are important — the care for a person who has recently developed confusion and that for someone with memory loss will be very different
- Always involve carers when assessing mental state.

Note: Impaired cognitive function following a hospital stay is closely associated with poor outcome.

Degree of mobility before fracture

Degree of mobility in older people is often more important than predicting outcomes for it can provide a baseline for goals and measurement of progress. Questions to ask include:

- How far could the patient walk before?
- What aids were required?
- Could the patient climb stairs?
- Did the patient become breathless after particular activities?

Consultation with someone who knows the patient often produces the most realistic and reliable results.

Functional ability

Questions on how the patient carries out daily living activities will enable a plan to be developed for when he or she is discharged. Patients should be asked questions on the following:

- Their normal daily routine
- Whether they can bath, wash and dress themselves without assistance
- If they are able to prepare and cook food themselves
- Their interests and hobbies
- Whether they can go out on their own to shop or visit friends. In some cases it may be relevant to ask whether they are in paid employment.

Social circumstance

The assessment should include questions about the following:

- The condition of the patient's home and ability to function in that environment
- Financial circumstances, including any problems with bills
- Support received from family, friends and others such as district nurses or home helps.

The discussion should include the individual's preferences for the future, the views of carers and relatives and what they think they can cope with realistically.

Source: Audit Commission (1995)

treatment were outlined in part one. An illustration of surgical fixation of a hip fracture is shown in Fig 2.

ACUTE WARD CARE AND ASSESSMENT

Most patients with hip fractures are older people and will require nursing care more in keeping with that given to patients in care of the elderly wards than those in orthopaedic wards. For example, many have hypertension, diabetes, dementia or Parkinson's disease.

These conditions are often associated with the fall that has resulted in the fracture. It is essential, though, that any medical conditions continue to be treated at the same time as care for the fracture is being given.

Assessment

Owing to the complex needs of these patients, a comprehensive assessment of their medical, nursing and social problems is essential. The assessment will be started in A&E and completed once the patient is in the acute ward.

The initial assessment in A&E will normally be for pressure sore risk, and key questions about the patient's social circumstances will be asked. Key information that should be obtained from an assessment is shown in Table 3.

REHABILITATION

Planning a rehabilitation programme involves nurses, surgeons, physiotherapists, occupational therapists and social workers. Nurses are central to the process because they are always present on the ward and can continue the work started by therapists and make sure that treatment plans are carried out and exercises are practised. Good nursing will tackle the problems of old age in a positive manner and encourage patients to be independent so they can return home.

For multidisciplinary working to be effective, one person should have responsibility for planning and review. The nurse is well placed to coordinate the various professional groups on a day-to-day basis and to liaise with the patient's family.

A collaborative approach to rehabilitation is not always realised owing to poor referral practices, failures in communication, poor service organisation, inadequate staff levels and problems in organising aids and appliances.

Pain control

Assessing pain used to be based on routines fixed to standard drug regimens but there are now a variety of pain assessment tools available which provide a more objective measure.

The value of multidisciplinary assessment and planning in the management of pain is well documented. Despite this it has been shown that nurses have mixed attitudes towards postoperative pain control and its assessment.

One study of RGNs in surgical units showed that although nurses appeared to be aware of the importance

Fig 2. Surgical fixation of a hip fracture: a surgical nail or screw stabilises the intertrochanteric fracture

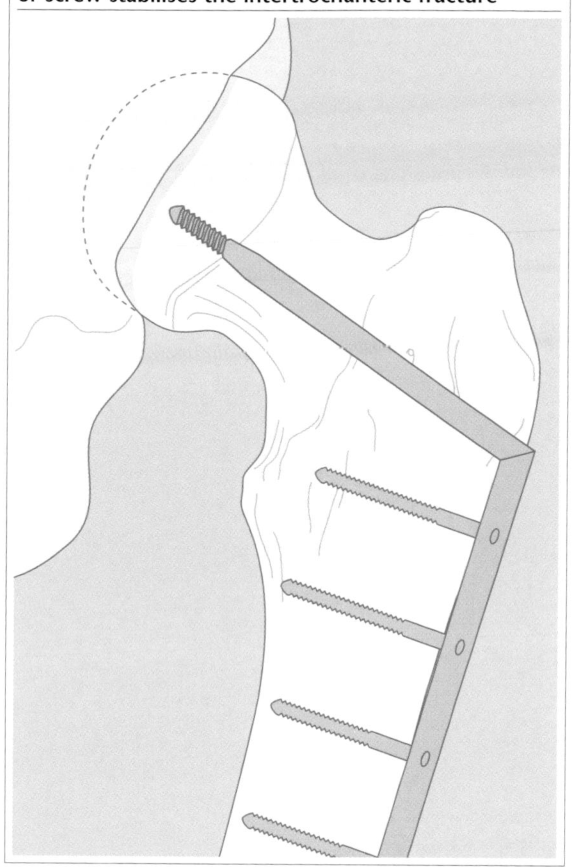

of accurate pain assessment and of managing it effectively, their attitudes were not always consistent with this (Thorn, 1997).

Timing of pain relief is important. Analgesia should be provided before procedures such as washing, turning and getting out of bed. Walking is especially difficult when in pain or when frightened of exacerbating pain.

A frequent criticism by physiotherapists is that patients are not given analgesia to fit with their physiotherapy times, with the result that they are in pain and unable to cooperate with their therapy (Audit Commission, 1995).

Promoting mobility

Early mobilisation reduces the risk of complications and also promote confidence (British Geriatric Society et al, 1987). The Royal College of Physicians' guidelines recommend that plans for the mobilisation, rehabilitation and discharge of patients should be made within four days of surgery, although in some units it is common for them to be mobilised the day after surgery.

Immobility can have serious consequences for older patients, causing pressure sores, deep vein thrombosis and pneumonia, all of which will prolong hospital stay and reduce the chance of the patient's returning to independent living.

An assessment of preoperative mobility will set a baseline for measuring progress and it is one of the most accurate predictors of recovery. Both should be an essential part of any multidisciplinary team's holistic plan of care.

Rehabilitation most commonly takes place in the orthopaedic ward although some hospitals have orthogeriatric units, general rehabilitation wards for the elderly and early support discharge or hospital-at-home schemes.

Whatever the setting a patient should be able to move around easily in an environment that has:

- Beds, chairs and toilets at the appropriate height
- Non-slip flooring
- Hand rails
- Good lighting
- Clear sign-posting of doors, toilets and bathrooms
- Easy access to spectacles, hearing- and walking aids
- Easy access to personal belongings.

Apart from the purely physical aspect of restoring a patient's mobility, the nurse working in a multidisciplinary team can do much to encourage independence and confidence.

Patients should be encouraged to dress and, ideally, wear their own clothes as well as take control over their daily activities such as choosing their food and eating it at a time of their choice.

New options for rehabilitation have emerged from changes in community care arrangements and are discussed in part three along with changes in the scope of practice for nurses.

THINKING POINT

- **In your experience, how effective is post-surgical pain relief? What strategies can help to ensure that analgesia is used to its best effect?**

PART THREE

Professional issues

Around 50–65% of patients with hip fracture regain their previous level of ambulation; 10–15% do not recover the ability to walk outside the home and are limited to household ambulation, while up to 20% because non-ambulatory (Koval et al, 1995). The ability to be able to walk has important implications, particularly for the elderly is they are to live independently.

Being able to go home after hospitalisation is an important outcome measure of fracture of the hip, and emphasis is being put on shorter hospital stays and early discharge. But research has shown that potentially this can have a negative effect on older patients who may have to cope on their own post-discharge (Fitzgerald et al, 1988). Therefore emphasis needs to be placed upon building strategies which take into account the special needs of older people.

The Department of Health has issued guidance on discharge policy both in the form of circulars (DoH, 1989) and a workbook (DoH, 1995). Further guidance has since been issued requiring health authorities to clarify responsibilities for continuing health care in an attempt to define more clearly when patients are ready for discharge (Audit Commission, 1995).

Discharge should be part of the planning process for rehabilitation. Patients can be assigned to a fast or slow stream rehabilitation programme which, as it progresses, allows a specific discharge date to be assigned and recorded in the notes.

Once a date has been specified, those responsible for post-discharge care should be alerted. Post-discharge care should be seen as a continuation of rehabilitation. In areas where there is a hospital-at-home or early support discharge scheme (see below), continuity of care tends to take place naturally, but in some areas where there is no such scheme, continuity of care may break down and the whole rehabilitation process may be compromised. This can mean that valuable progress gained during rehabilitation is lost, and may even result in a patient's being admitted to residential care or to a nursing home instead of to his/her own home.

A study of discharge planning after hip fracture (Audit Commission, 1995), looking at 360 patient notes from nine hospitals, found little evidence of effective planning. Despite hospitals being required to draw up and carry out planned discharge procedures, only a quarter contained a record of the anticipated discharge date and only a similar proportion contained any assessment of primary health care services. According to the study, factors which contributed to this were:

- Little awareness of any discharge policy by nurses and social workers
- Few formal planning meetings, with multidisciplinary working taking place only during ward rounds, which is inconvenient for staff who are not ward-based such as therapists and social workers
- A lack of particular training on discharge policy for nurses or social workers — nurses were therefore unfamiliar with how to refer to social services and social

workers said the focus of any training they had was only on form-filling, not practicalities
- Poor monitoring of discharge, unclear responsibilities, and reasons for readmission of patients rarely monitored.

The Audit Commission, however, has acknowledged the dilemma faced by hospital staff who are under constant pressure to discharge patients and by social workers who have to tailor individual care within limited budgets, seeing these as a major impediment to improving discharge procedures.

A multidisciplinary approach to care, provided by health-care workers working closely together, may be an effective way to improve short- and long-term outcomes for patients with hip fracture. The following health-care professionals should be involved in the formulation of a hospital's discharge procedure:
- Ward nurses
- Community nurses
- Therapists
- General managers from the appropriate clinical directorate
- A community development manager
- A social services manager and a hospital social worker
- A representative from the community health council
- GP/hospital medical staff.

Several studies have documented the short-term efficacy of multidisciplinary working with the use of appropriate care maps linked to medical and nursing protocols: fewer postoperative complications, fewer transfers to intensive care, improved ambulation on discharge and reduced rate of discharge to nursing homes have all been demonstrated (Ogilvie-Harris, 1993). However, although a case management approach to care after discharge may reduce the overall need for care when at home, mortality, status on discharge and level of functional recovery have been shown to remain the same as for patients receiving standard care (Jette et al, 1987).

DISCHARGE LIAISON NURSES

Discharge liaison nurses provide a link between hospital and community. Their main role is to attend discharge planning meetings and to familiarise themselves with the needs of individual patients. However, unless there are sufficient discharge nurses in one hospital, they may well find it difficult to cover a whole hospital effectively. The use of discharge liaison nurses may also mean that ward nurses become unfamiliar with local services. It has been suggested that a more useful role for these nurses would be for them to establish frameworks for liaison between services and facilitate the setting up of arrangements between ward and community staff.

EARLY SUPPORTED DISCHARGE

Hospitals-at-home and early discharge schemes can now offer real advantages for patients who are well enough, allowing them to learn how to cope in their own surroundings. Such schemes can ensure not only that rehabilitation is suited to individual needs but also can enable a smooth handover between hospital and community staff.

Hospital-at-home schemes in particular have become more popular over the past five years, partly to reduce lengths of stay in hospital and partly because purchasers and providers have been keen to shift the balance of care over into the community.

For hip fracture patients a hospital-at-home scheme offers them:
- Discharge soon after surgery
- Assessment by a district nurse
- Support related to needs — some schemes offer, initially, 24-hour nursing care
- Physiotherapy
- Occupational therapy
- Patient aids.

Whether hospital-at-home schemes are cost-effective has been a matter of controversy, but it is now thought that they cost less than inpatient care for hip fracture patients, although it is emphasised that such schemes work properly only when they are adequately funded (Hollingworth et al, 1993).

CASE MANAGEMENT/MANAGED CARE

Case management has been used by health and social work professionals for many years as a way of coordinating the care of clients with complex needs but their use has been expanding over the past decade (Laxade and Hale, 1995).

Older patients with a fractured neck of femur are a good example of the type of client group that can benefit from managed care systems which aim to connect previously unconnected or poorly connected parts of a health-care system, for example hospital services with community services or in-patient care with outpatient care.

The model demands the appointment of a case manager or fitting a case management role into an existing post. In acute care, nurses have increasingly been seen as the most appropriate professionals to carry out this role.

Case management uses care maps and variance management to organise care and provide a framework for planning care linked to expected outcomes. The maps are multidisciplinary and flexible enough to incorporate advances in care as well as being used to carry out clinical audit.

The case manager is responsible for coordinating the activities of the care map and so must be given authority to extend his/her influence beyond the confines of a particular setting.

LITIGATION AND DOCUMENTATION

Orthopaedic nurses are increasingly being asked to act as expert witnesses in litigation cases. Although specific complaints about nursing care are uncommon, the number of patients taking legal action against their health-care providers is expected to continue to increase (Lord, 1995). The *Patient's Charter* has given the public information on the standards of care they can expect to receive.

The legal profession is starting to realise that although doctors can provide an expert opinion on medical care, they are not always the most appropriate professional to comment on other aspects of care (Prior, 1997).

In orthopaedics, a specialist nurse, physiotherapist or occupational therapist may well be the most knowledgeable person.

The preparation of any legal case will involve the detailed scrutiny of patient records, witness and client statements. It is here that the care plan can be vital. Completed at the time of admission it can identify the needs or problems of patients as they track through the hospital. But it is often never referred to again after admission or added to or evaluated, although some areas use an evaluation sheet or progress sheet to chart a patient's progress. However, these may not be included in the patient records, meaning that much of the information about the nursing care given to a particular patient may be missing.

An Audit Commission report (1992) demonstrated that standards of care planning and record-keeping were generally poor, although this is often because of staff shortages. If this is the case it is recommended that such shortages are documented, although this may be difficult in practice owing to fears of recrimination.

Table 4. Ways managers and clinicians can improve the care of patients with fractured neck of femur (RCP, 1989)

Managers and clinicians should:

- Allocate responsibility for reviewing services, producing a strategy and monitoring standards of care and outcome
- Review mortality and morbidity annually
- Undertake studies to investigate different management strategies
- Ensure that patients spend no more than one hour in A&E
- Include assessment of co-existing medical problems, mental function and social circumstances in pre-operative planning
- Begin discharge planning at the assessment stage
- Ensure operations are carried out within 24 hours by senior staff
- Make plans for mobilisation, rehabilitation and discharge or transfer within four days of the operation
- Ensure close working relationships between orthopaedic surgeons and geriatricians
- Make available experienced nurses, physiotherapy and occupational therapy services
- Provide a means of liaison with community services and carers.

FUTURE CHANGES IN PRACTICES

The increasing incidence of hip fracture is likely to be a continuing problem for the NHS partly because of the increasing number of patients but also because of the increasing age and frailty of those people fracturing their hips.

It has been projected that in England alone, the population aged 65 or older will rise 11% between 1991 and 2011 and it has been estimated that the number of patients admitted to hospital with a fractured hip will rise 22% to 68,894 by 2011 (Hollingworth et al, 1995). This increasing strain could be countered in the continued improvement of rehabilitative and surgical techniques, allowing early return of mobility and discharge, but as significant reductions in length of stay have already been made (see part one), any further improvements would have to be substantial. It is thought, however, that such a reduction, on top of those already made, is not feasible (Laxade and Hall, 1995).

Any innovation in acute hospital treatment, whether surgical or rehabilitative, would have implications for non-acute services, community services and families of patients. Alternatively, prevention schemes could be directed at the incidence of hip fracture, with the aim of reversing the current trend.

A review of preventive measures concluded that increased physical activity and the cessation of smoking could have a major effect on the incidence of bone fracture, either in terms of increasing bone mass at a younger age or of reducing loss of bone and maintaining structure (Law et al, 1991).

There is continued debate over the cost-effectiveness of hormone replacement therapy as a prevention strategy and further studies into the issues are needed (Goddard, 1990). Osteoporosis is another issue in prevention and the role of drugs has again been controversial. Only one treatment, alendronate, has been shown actually to reduce the risk of hip fracture (Black et al, 1997). In that study, the treatment was not associated with a difference in the rate of adverse effects compared to placebo and it has been suggested that the treatment could reduce the consequences of osteoporosis in high-risk women.

Another modifiable risk factor is the fall that causes the fracture, the challenge being not only to understand what causes a fall but also to find out whether behaviour and environment can be modified to reduce incidence and impact. It is generally accepted that exercise programmes to improve physical fitness, agility and speed of response of older people are useful as a preventive measure, but, on the other hand, one study has shown that increased activity can be associated with an increased risk of falling (Campbell et al, 1990).

Modifying the environment of an older person can also be considered, but again the benefits are not always straightforward, with one study suggesting that some interventions are actually increasing the risk of injury (Gibson et al, 1987).

Proving the cost-effectiveness of preventive strategies and then implementing them, together with improved acute, non-acute and community care for those who have fractured their hip, could help avoid the 'worst-case' scenario of the NHS in England alone having to cope with 254,720 cases by 2031 (Hollingworth et al, 1995).

Whatever their cause, hip fracture poses an important challenge to purchasers and providers over the coming decades and professional bodies such as the Royal College of Physicians have already made their recommendations about how managers and clinicians can improve the care of these patients (see Table 4). Either extra hospital beds or major initiatives will be needed to prevent fracture, improve treatment and provide for community care.

REFERENCES

Anderson, G.H. et al (1993) The incidence of proximal fractures in an English county. *Journal of Bone and Joint Surgery*; 75(b): 441–444.

Audit Commission (1992) *The Virtue of Patients: Making Best Use of Ward Resources*. London: HMSO.

Audit Commission (1995) *United They Stand: Coordinating Care for Elderly Patients with Hip Fracture*. London: HMSO.

Black, D.M. et al (1997) Randomised trial of effect of alendronate on risk of fracture in women with existing vertebral fractures. *Lancet*; 348: 1535–1541.

Campbell, A.J. et al (1990) Circumstances and consequences of falls experienced by a community population 70 years and over during a prospective study. *Age and Ageing*; 19: 136–141.

Department of Health (1989) *Hospital Discharge Workbook: A Manual on Hospital Discharge Practice*. London: DoH.

Department of Health (1995) *NHS Responsibilities for Meeting Continuing Health Needs*. London: DoH.

Department of Health. (1989) *Hospital In-patient Inquiry: In-Patient and Day-Case Trends, 1979–1985*. London: HMSO.

Fitzgerald, J.F. et al (1988) The care of elderly patients with hip fracture: Changes since the implementation of the prospective payment system. *New England Journal of Medicine;* 319: 1392–1397.

Gibson, J. et al (1987) The prevention of falls in later life. *Danish Medical Bulletin*; 34: S4, 1-24.

Goddard, M. (1990) *The Cost-effectiveness of Hormone Replacement Therapy: A Review. Discussion Paper 73*. York: Centre for Health Economics, Health Economics Consortium, University of York.

Hollingworth, W. et al (1993) Cost analysis of early discharge after hip fracture. *British Medical Journal*; 307: 903–906.

Hollingworth, W. et al (1995) The cost of treating hip fractures in the twenty-first century. *Journal of Public Health Medicine*; 17: 3, 269–276.

Jette, A.M. et al (1987) Functional recovery after hip fracture. *Archives of Practical Medical Rehabilitation*; 68: 735–740.

Koval, K.J.et al (1995)Ambulatory ability after hip fracture: A prospective study in geriatric patients. *Clinical Orthopaedics*; 310: 150–159.

Law, M.R. et al (1991) Strategies for prevention of osteoporosis and hip fracture. *British Medical Journal;* 303: 453–459.

Laxade, S., Hale, C.A. (1995) Managed care 2: an opportunity for nursing. *British Journal of Nursing;* 4: 6, 345–350.

Lord, J. (1995) Expert witness survey — the results. *Your Witness*; 1 (September).

Lufkin, E.G. et al (1992) Treatment of postmenopausal osteoporosis with transdermal estrogen. *Annals of Internal Medicine*; 117: 1–9.

Office of Population Censuses and Surveys (1993) *National Population Projections, 1991-Based*. London: HMSO.

Ogilvie-Harris, D.J. et al (1993) Elderly patients with hip fractures: improved outcome with the use of care maps with high-quality medical and nursing protocols. *Journal of Orthopaedic Trauma*; 7: 428–437.

Overgaard, K. et al (1992) Effect of calcitonin given intranasally on bone mass and fracture rates in established osteoporosis: a dose response study. *British Medical Journal*; 305: 556–561.

Pak, C.Y. et al. Treatment of post-menopausal osteoporosis with slow release sodium fluoride. *Annals of Internal Medicine*; 123: 401–408.

Pellino, T.A. (1994) How to manage hip fractures. *American Journal of Nursing*; 94: 46–50.

Prior, M. (1997) The case for the orthopaedic nurse expert. *The Journal of Orthopaedic Nursing*; 1: 67–70.

Royal College of Physicians (1989) *Fractured Neck of Femur: Prevention and Management*. London: RCP.

Spector, T.D. et al (1990) Trends in admissions for hip fracture in England and Wales, 1968 to 1985. *British Medical Journal*; 300: 1173–1174.

Storm, T. et al. (1990) Effect of intermittent cyclical etidronate therapy on bone mass and fracture rate in women with postmenopausal osteoporosis. *New England Journal of Medicine;* 322: 1265–1271.

The British Geriatrics Society et al (1987) *Improving the Care of Elderly People in Hospital*. London: RCN.

Thorn, M. (1997) A survey of nurses' attitudes towards the assessment and control of postoperative pain. *Journal of Orthopaedic Nursing*; 1: 30–38.

Thromboembolic Risk Factors (THRIFT) Consensus Group (1992) Risk of and prophylaxis for venous thromboembolism in hospital patients. *British Medical Journal*; 302: 567–574.

Tilyard, M.Wet al (1992) Treatment of postmenopausal osteoporosis with calcitriol or calcium. *New England Journal of Medicine*; 326: 357–362.

Todd, C.J. et al (1995) Differences in mortality after fracture of the hip: The East Anglian audit. *British Medical Journal*; 310: 904–908.

Useful addresses

Age Concern England (The National Council on Ageing)
Astral House
1268 London Road
London SW16 4ER
0181 765 7200

National Osteoporosis Society
PO Box 10
Radstock
Bath
Avon BA3 3YB
01761 471771

Fractured neck of femur

Assessment

When you have read the unit and completed any further reading, you can use the questions below to test your understanding of the topic. Answers can be found on the next page.

1. Of those who fracture their hips, what percentage will die?:

- [ ] 1 5%
- [ ] 2 10%
- [ ] 3 15%
- [ ] 4 20%

2. The most common underlying pathology of hip fracture is:

- [ ] 1 Dementia
- [ ] 2 Parkinson's disease
- [ ] 3 Osteoporosis
- [ ] 4 Bone cancer

3. A subcapital fracture is:

- [ ] 1 A fracture through the middle of the neck of the femur
- [ ] 2 A fracture through the base of the neck of the femur
- [ ] 3 An extracapsular fracture
- [ ] 4 A fracture distal to the articular margin of the femur head

4. Internal fixation is most suitable for:

- [ ] 1 Any type of hip fracture
- [ ] 2 A large, basal fracture
- [ ] 3 A fracture to the subtrochanteric region
- [ ] 4 A fracture to the intertrochanteric region

5. Anticoagulant prophylaxis with warfarin or dextran prevents what percentage of deep vein thrombi:

- [ ] 1 20–30%
- [ ] 2 30–40%
- [ ] 3 40–50%
- [ ] 4 50–60%

6. It has been recommended that patients with hip fracture should not spend any longer than one hour in A&E because:

- [ ] 1 Surgery must be carried out within 12 hours of sustaining the fracture
- [ ] 2 Patients are likely to have spent a long time at home before being discovered
- [ ] 3 Patients are likely to be in a confused state
- [ ] 4 Patients are likely to be dehydrated

7. Withholding food and water before surgery has been shown to be sufficient for:

- [ ] 1 Four hours
- [ ] 2 Eight hours
- [ ] 3 Twelve hours
- [ ] 4 Fifteen hours

8. Assessing how mobile a patient was before fracture is useful as:

- [ ] 1 A guide for physiotherapy teams
- [ ] 2 An indicator for social services deciding whether to make any modification to a patient's home
- [ ] 3 An accurate predictor of recovery
- [ ] 4 A measure of the success of surgical fixation

9. Continuity of care is less likely to break down in hospital-at-home schemes because:

- [ ] 1 Discharge policy is more likely to be adhered to
- [ ] 2 The community staff are more likely to have had specific training
- [ ] 3 They are linked, and have often grown out of existing systems of care
- [ ] 4 An outreach nurse retains care of each patient

10. Royal College of Physicians guidelines recommend that plans for mobilisation, rehabilitation and discharge should be made within:

- [ ] 1 A week of admission
- [ ] 2 A week of surgery
- [ ] 3 A day of admission
- [ ] 4 Four days of surgery

11 **Many drug treatments have been shown to increase bone mass but only one has been proven to reduce actual risk of fracture. It is:**

- [ ] 1 Calcitonin
- [ ] 2 Bisphosphonate
- [ ] 3 Oestrogen
- [ ] 4 Alendronate

12 **Impaired cognitive function in older patients with hip fracture is:**

- [ ] 1 Associated with an increased likelihood of a fall occurring
- [ ] 2 Likely to affect the choice between prosthetic replacement and surgical fixation
- [ ] 3 Associated with poor outcome after discharge
- [ ] 4 Associated with an increased likelihood of early supported discharge

ANSWERS

Fractured neck of femur

1: Of those who fracture their hips, what percentage will die?
3) 15%

2: The most common underlying pathology of hip fracture is:
3) Osteoporosis

3: A subcapital fracture is:
4) A fracture distal to the articular margin of the femur head

4: Internal fixation is most suitable for:
1) Any type of hip fracture

5: Anticoagulant prophylaxis with warfarin or dextran prevents what percentage of deep vein thrombi:
3) 40–50%

6: It has been recommended that patients with hip fracture should not spend any longer than one hour in A&E because:
2) Patients are likely to have spent a long time at home before being discovered

7: Withholding food and water before surgery has been shown to be sufficient for:
1) Four hours

8: Assessing how mobile a patient was before fracture is useful as:
3) An accurate predictor of recovery

9: Continuity of care is less likely to break down in hospital-at-home schemes because:
3) They are linked, and have often grown out of existing systems of care

10: Royal College of Physicians guidelines recommend that plans for mobilisation, rehabilitation and discharge should be made within:
4) Four days of surgery

11: Many drug treatments have been shown to increase bone mass but only one has been proven to reduce actual risk of fracture. It is:
4) Alendronate

12: Impaired cognitive function in older patients with hip fracture is:
1) Associated with an increased likelihood of a fall occurring

Medication

Knowledge for practice

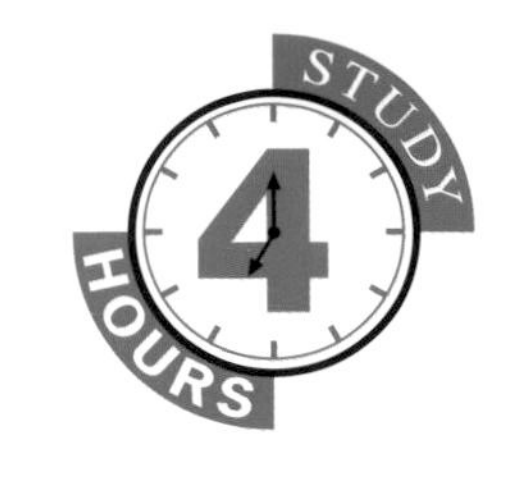

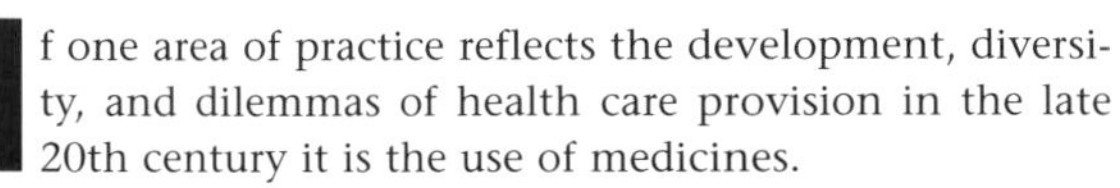

If one area of practice reflects the development, diversity, and dilemmas of health care provision in the late 20th century it is the use of medicines.

Over the 50-year history of the NHS the evolution of modern pharmacotherapy has transformed the treatment and prevention of ill health in the UK almost beyond recognition. Yet, such development has not been without cost, both to health care organisations and to the patients they aim to care for.

With an ever increasing number of medicines has come an inevitable increase in the amount of resources consumed by drug treatments and a proportionate rise in the expectations of patients as to what such medicines can achieve in improving their health.

Concerns have also grown as to the robustness of the evidence base on which much drug treatment is constructed, and the potential harm that medicines may cause.

For practitioners involved in the provision of health care, the administration of medicines is arguably the only major clinical intervention that consistently links patients under their care irrespective of the cause of their illness. Yet such is the pace of development of modern medicines that there are increasing numbers of pitfalls for the unwary practitioner.

The clinical and legislative principles that underpin the safe and effective use of medicines in hospitals, in nursing homes and in the community are complex and confusing and are in parts failing to reflect the needs of modern clinical practice.

The aim here is to offer guidance to nurses on how best to navigate the medicines minefield.

PHARMACOLOGY

The effects of drugs on the body (pharmacodynamics) and the effects of the body on a drug over time (pharmacokinetics) are considered in the science of pharmacology.

It is developments in the field of pharmacology that have led to most of the significant developments in drug treatment of the past 50 years, for example, histamine antagonists, beta-blockers and so on.

While an in-depth appreciation of clinical pharmacology is not essential to safe drug use it is important for practitioners to possess a basic understanding of how a drug might be expected to exert its action once given. Moreover, such an understanding offers insight into how the effects of drugs might be experienced by the patient, and also the extent to which undesirable effects may be produced.

How drugs work

The vast majority of drugs produce their effects by reacting with specific protein molecules in the cell membrane. These cells are called receptors.

Such receptors are normally responsive to chemical stimuli produced by the body, for example, neurotransmitters or hormones.

Drugs may mimic the body's natural stimuli and thereby act as agonists, or may inhibit them, thereby acting as blockers to 'normal' physiological responses or antagonists. Some examples of drugs and their modes of action are listed in Table 1.

Those drugs that do not act directly on receptor sites may act principally via one of the following mechanisms:

- Enzyme inhibition, for example warfarin
- Enzyme activation, for example thrombolytic agents used after myocardial infarction
- Inhibition of cellular transport processes, for example calcium channel blockers and diuretics
- Action by chemicophysical properties of the drug, for example osmotic laxatives
- Most anti-infective drugs (for example, antibiotics, antivirals) act by inhibiting biochemical processes that are unique to the target organism (for example, bacteria).

The extent to which a drug reacts selectively with different receptors defines how specific its actions are, and this in turn may determine how extensively its actions, both desirable and undesirable, are felt throughout the body. For example, the beta-blocker propranolol is not selective for the adrenergic receptors in the heart. Therefore it exerts an effect on other physiological systems that are under adrenergic control. For example, the bronchi-

Table 1. Mode of action of a range of drugs

Drug	*Indication*	*Mode of action*
Cimetidine	Ulcer healing	Blocks histamine receptors in parietal cells
Fluoxetine (Prozac)	Depression	Blocks serotonin uptake at the nerve endings
Salbutamol	Asthma	Stimulates adrenergic receptors in the lung
Morphine	Pain relief	Stimulates opioid receptors in the central nervous system
Allopurinol	Gout	Inhibits uric acid-forming enzyme

oles may be constricted. Conversely the selective beta-blocker atenolol has a much greater degree of selectivity for receptors in the heart, and therefore is much less likely to cause bronchospasm.

The reaction of the drug with its receptor site is not a guarantee that an immediate therapeutic response will be generated. The speed of onset of the drug depends on what other pharmacological and physiological stages have to be translated before a therapeutic effect can be realised, and this varies enormously between drugs. For example, the administration of salbutamol into the lung produces a more or less immediate bronchodilation.

Similarly, the use of sublingual glyceryl trinitrate produces a rapid vasodilation thereby reducing the symptoms of angina. Conversely, the symptomatic relief of depression may take up to three weeks when treated with an antidepressant such as fluoxetine (Prozac).

For a drug to achieve its therapeutic effect, however, it must not only reach its site of action, but it must be present in a sufficiently high concentration and for a sufficient length of time. If either of these criteria is not met, then the effects of the drug will be subtherapeutic.

The way in which a drug behaves in the body over time is described by its pharmacokinetic profile. This profile describes the way in which the drug is absorbed, distributed, metabolised and excreted by the body once it has been administered.

These parameters are responsible for determining a great many of the practicalities of drug administration. For example, how well the drug is absorbed via the gastrointestinal tract will determine whether or not it can be formulated as a tablet or capsule.

The rate at which the drug is metabolised and excreted will determine how often it needs to be administered and, if being given intravenously, whether or not it can be given by a direct injection or as an infusion.

In older patients, age-related reductions in hepatic and renal function mean that dose reductions must be made to many drugs to prevent toxicity from occurring.

For the small number of drugs with narrow margins between optimal and suboptimal dosing, the so-called narrow therapeutic index (for example, phenytoin, gentamicin) detailed pharmacokinetic profiling forms an essential feature of their safe and effective use.

While the majority of drugs in use today are administered by mouth, this route of administration is arguably the least reliable in terms of delivering the drug to the intended site of action.

A number of factors may act singly or in combination to significantly reduce the amount of drug absorbed via the gastrointestinal tract into the systemic circulation. These include:

- The effect of gastric motility. In patients in whom the rate of gastric emptying is increased, drug absorption will be reduced
- The existence of a malabsorption syndrome: for example, Crohn's or coeliac disease may decrease or in some instances increase drug absorption
- The effect of gastric pH. Some drugs are particularly sensitive to the acidic environment of the stomach and may be degraded before significant absorption can occur
- Food. Many drugs undergo a physicochemical reaction in the presence of food, which reduces their absorption.

Drug formulation

In many instances the formulation of a drug offers a means by which shortcomings in the pharmacokinetic profile may be overcome.

In the majority of such cases formulation is used to increase the amount of drug likely to reach the intended site of action. For example, many of the drugs used in the treatment of asthma are suitable for administration by mouth, but to achieve therapeutically active concentrations in the lung would require very large doses to be given. This would increase the risk of side-effects and may make treatment difficult for patients to tolerate.

By formulating the drugs as aerosols they can be administered directly into the lung, thereby achieving high concentrations at the desired site of action, and reducing the risk of side-effects by avoiding the drugs' entry into the systemic circulation.

In recent years pharmaceutical manufacturers have increasingly used the transdermal route as means of delivering drugs into the systemic circulation.

Many patients now receive their daily doses of antianginals, hormone replacement therapy and nicotine replacement therapy through a stick-on patch that delivers a constant amount of drug through the skin over a 12- or 24-hour period.

Formulation may also be used to extend the duration of action of a drug by modifying the rate at which it is absorbed into the systemic circulation.

Such modifications are usually used to reduce the number of doses that have to be given each day. For example the development of modified release formulations of morphine have made it possible to reduce the routine dose interval from every four hours or six times a day to twice a day.

Such developments can have a significant influence on a patient's attitude toward their drug therapy (see part three).

ADVERSE DRUG REACTIONS

While the development of modern pharmacotherapy has brought about enormous changes to the way in which ill health is managed, the use of medicines to bring about health gain is not without risk.

Indeed, the decision to use medicines to treat or prevent ill health is very much a matter of balancing risk and benefit.

Such decisions need to take account of the efficacy of the drug, the likelihood of adverse reactions developing as

Fig 1. How reduced liver and kidney function can affect drug absorption

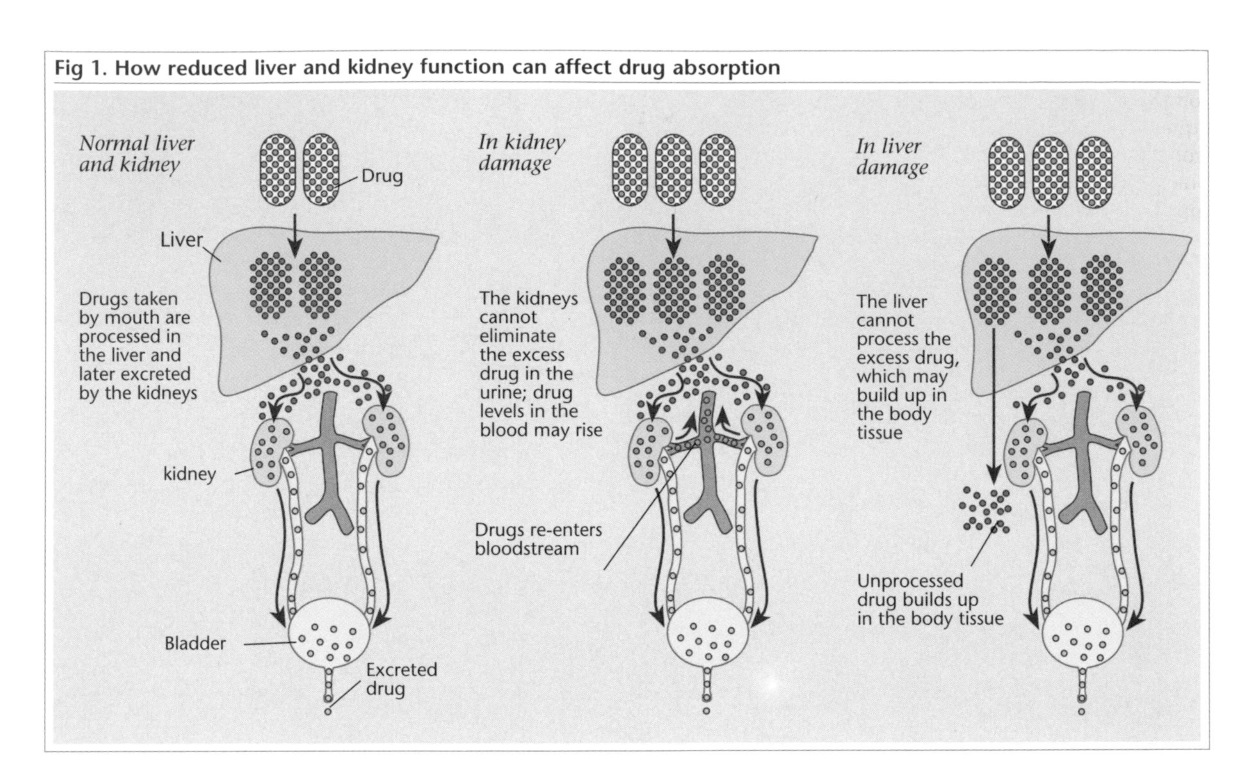

a consequence of its use and their potential seriousness. Similarly the possibility of interaction occurring with other drugs requires careful consideration.

Types of adverse reaction

An adverse reaction to a drug is any response to the drug that is unintended, and of no benefit to the patient. They may be related to the normal pharmacological action of the drug, so-called type A or augmented reactions. These reactions are related to the dose of the drug and can usually be predicted from the drug's pharmacological profile.

Such reactions include the anticholinergic effects of antidepressants such as amitriptyline that cause a dry mouth or urinary retention, and the drowsiness caused by drugs such diazepam.

Reactions that are unrelated to the drug's conventional pharmacology are described as type B or bizarre reactions. These are usually unrelated to the dose administered and are unpredictable.

Such reactions include anaphylaxis to penicillins. The morbidity associated with adverse reactions to drugs is undoubtedly significant.

Adverse reactions are thought to occur in as many as 20% of hospital inpatients and are thought to be responsible for up to 4% of hospital admissions.

There are some groups of patients in whom the risk of adverse reaction is known to be higher — for example, in pregnancy or breast-feeding mothers. But this relates in particular to older patients, in whom age-related changes in drug handling (for example, reductions in liver and renal function, see Fig 1) combine with the existence of multiple pathologies significantly to increase the risk of adverse reaction.

Such risk is compounded by the use in older patients of many drugs that are known to be associated with a high incidence of adverse reactions, such as those acting on the cardiovascular and central nervous systems.

Clearly, such considerations require diligence on the part of practitioners when reviewing the overall benefits of initiating drug treatment.

INTERACTIONS

For older patients the risks of drug treatment are not solely related to the possibility of adverse reaction occurring.

As the highest consumers of medicines (in the UK patients over 65 consume 43% of all prescribed medicines), they are also particularly at risk of problems associated with drug interactions.

A drug interaction is said to occur when the effects of one drug are altered by the effects of another. Such interaction usually results in an adverse drug reaction.

The mechanisms by which interactions occur are complex but are summarised into three basic types:

- Those relating to physicochemical reaction between wo drugs: for example, mixing the antibiotic gentamicin with heparin in the same syringe or intravenous line
- Those relating to alterations in a drugs pharmacokinetic profile: for example, carbamazepine increases the metabolism of oestrogens contained in the oral

contraceptive thereby reducing its effectiveness

- Interactions altering the effect of a drugs at its site of action: for example, the administration of naloxone to a patient who has received morphine, will result in the effects of the morphine being reversed as naloxone displaces it from is receptor.

CONCLUSION

Medication is a mainstay of the treatment offered by health services. However, effective treatment is influenced by a broad range of factors. Understanding these factors supports the nurse's role in ensuring that drug therapy is as effective as possible.

THINKING POINTS

- **In your clinical area, how far do considerations of pharmacodynamics influence the administration of drugs?**
- **What measures could be taken to ensure that drugs are given at the most appropriate time?**

PART TWO

Administration of medicines

There are two main factors that determine whether or not a drug will reach its intended site of action in the body.

These are:

- The bioavailaibility of the drug
- How the drug is given.

BIOAVAILAIBILITY

As described in part one, the extent to which a drug is present in the body in sufficiently high concentrations to exert a therapeutic effect is largely a consequence of its bioavailaibility.

This term describes that proportion of an administered drug that reaches the systemic circulation and is therefore available for distribution to the intended site of action.

Drugs that are given by direct intravenous (IV) injection have 100% bioavailability. Some drugs that are particularly well absorbed by the gastrointestinal mucosa may have bioavailability comparable to that of an intravenous dose: for example, the antibiotic ciprofloxacin. Most drugs, however do not and hence the dose given orally is usually higher than that given parenterally.

The bioavailability of a drug can clearly be influenced by the route of administration and therefore its formulation.

The various routes of administration available have advantages and disadvantages associated with them.

ROUTES OF DRUG ADMINISTRATION

All the routes for drug administration need to be understood in term of their implications for the effectiveness of the drug therapy and the patient's experience.

Oral administration

While by far the most frequently used route of drug administration, the oral route is problematic because of the unpredictable nature of gastro-intestinal drug absorption; also the extent to which patients can tolerate solid dose forms, that is, tablets and capsules.

This may be particularly relevant in the very young and older patients. In such cases the use of liquids or soluble formulations may be helpful. Many drugs, however, are not sufficiently stable in solution for liquid formulation to be made viable, and in such cases careful consideration should be given to the options of switching to alternative drug treatment.

Such difficulties frequently arise in patients receiving 'modified release' preparations.

Sublingual

The sublingual mucosa offers a rich supply of blood vessels through which drugs can be absorbed. While not a common route of drug administration, it offers rapid absorption into the systemic circulation and avoidance of the so-called 'first pass effect'.

This occurs when certain drugs administered orally and absorbed via the gastrointestinal tract may be metabolised extensively by passing directly through the mesenteric circulation, thereby reducing their bioavailaibility.

The most common example of sublingual administration is glyceryl trinitrate in the treatment of acute angina.

Recognising the difficulty that many patients experience when swallowing tablets, however, the pharmaceutical industry has increasingly begun to formulate and market wafer-based versions of tablets that dissolve rapidly under the tongue.

Such presentations are being aimed at particular markets, such as the treatment of migraine and pain.

Rectal administration

While the rectal route has considerable disadvantages in terms of patient acceptability (in the UK at least) and predictability, it does offer a number of benefits.

It offers a valuable means of localised drug delivery into the large bowel: for example, the use of rectal steroids in the form of enemas or suppositories in the treatment of colitis.

It can also be used to circumvent problems of nausea

and vomiting which mitigate against use of the oral route: for example, administration of antiemetics.

Topical administration

In the management of localised disease the direct application of medicines has obvious advantages. The chosen drug can be made available almost directly at the intended site of action, and because the systemic circulation is not reached, the risk of systemic side effects is reduced.

Examples of such administration are many, for example, the use of eye drops containing beta-blockers in the treatment of glaucoma, the application of topical steroids in the management of dermatitis, the use of inhalers containing bronchodilators in the treatment of asthma, and the use of pessaries containing clotrimazole in the treatment of vaginal candidiasis.

The topical administration of medicines has, however, also become a popular way of getting drugs into the systemic circulation through the skin. The development of drug containing transdermal patches started with the introduction of a product for the treatment of nausea in the early 1980s.

The market for such products has since grown to include a wide range of disease management areas including, the prophylaxis of angina (glyceryl trinitrate), the treatment of chronic pain (fentanyl) and hormone replacement (oestrogens).

While the use of transdermal drug administration is not without its problems, for example some preparations can cause local skin reactions, many patients find it a welcome alternative to taking tablets.

Intramuscular and subcutaneous injection (Fig 2 and 3)

In general the injection of drugs into the muscle or the adipose tissue beneath the skin allows a deposit or 'depot' of drug to be established that will be released gradually into the systemic circulation over a period of time.

By altering the formulation of the drug, the period over which it is released can be influenced. For example, the formulation of antipsychotic agents such as flupenthixol in oil allows them to be administered on a monthly or three-monthly basis.

Similarly, by changing the extent to which insulin is crystallised, its duration of action can be varied from very short (Actrapid) to very long (ultralente).

IV injection

In many ways the administration of medicines via the intravenous route is an admission that the use of other routes will not allow for an intended therapeutic outcome to be met.

Not only is the IV route inconvenient for patient and practitioner alike, but it carries arguably the greatest risk of any route of drug administration. By administering directly into the systemic circulation either by direct injection of infusion the drug is instantaneously distributed to its sites of action.

Such administration is frequently complex and confusing. It may require dose calculations to be made, dilutions to be carried out, information to be gathered on administration rates and compatabilities with other IV solutions, and increasingly frequently, the use of technically advanced programmable infusion devices.

Moreover, the preparation of IV medicines requires the use of aseptic technique, often in a ward environment that is wholly unsuited to such work.

It is imperative that practitioners involved in such drug administration can demonstrate their competence to prac-

Fig 2. Intramuscular injection technique

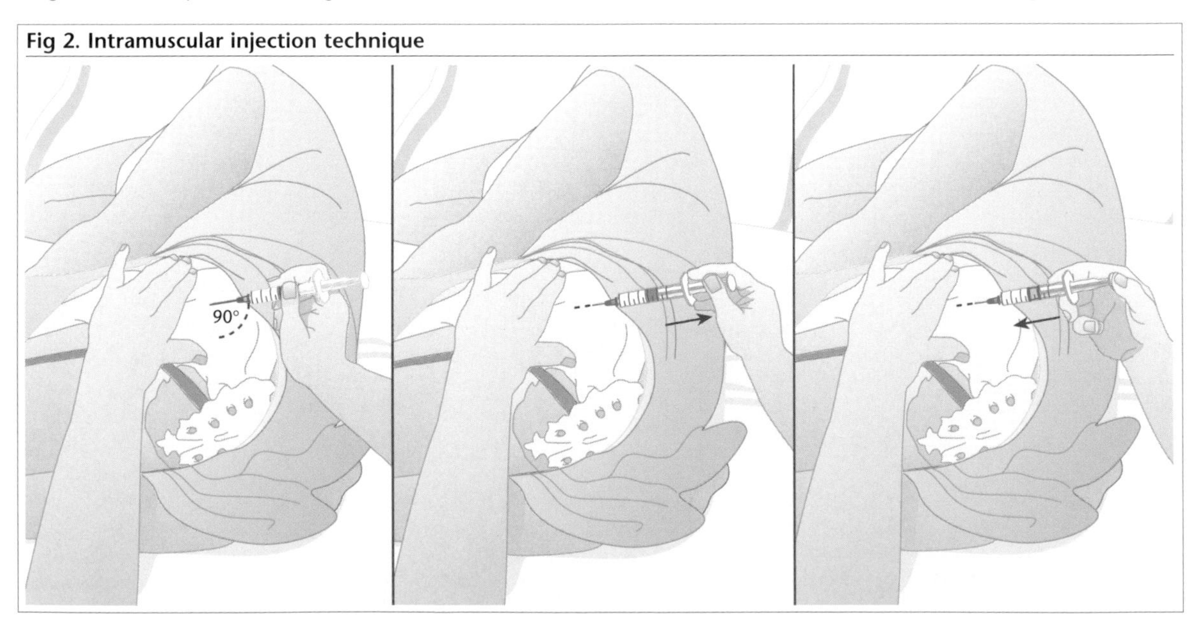

Fig 3. Subcutaneous injection technique

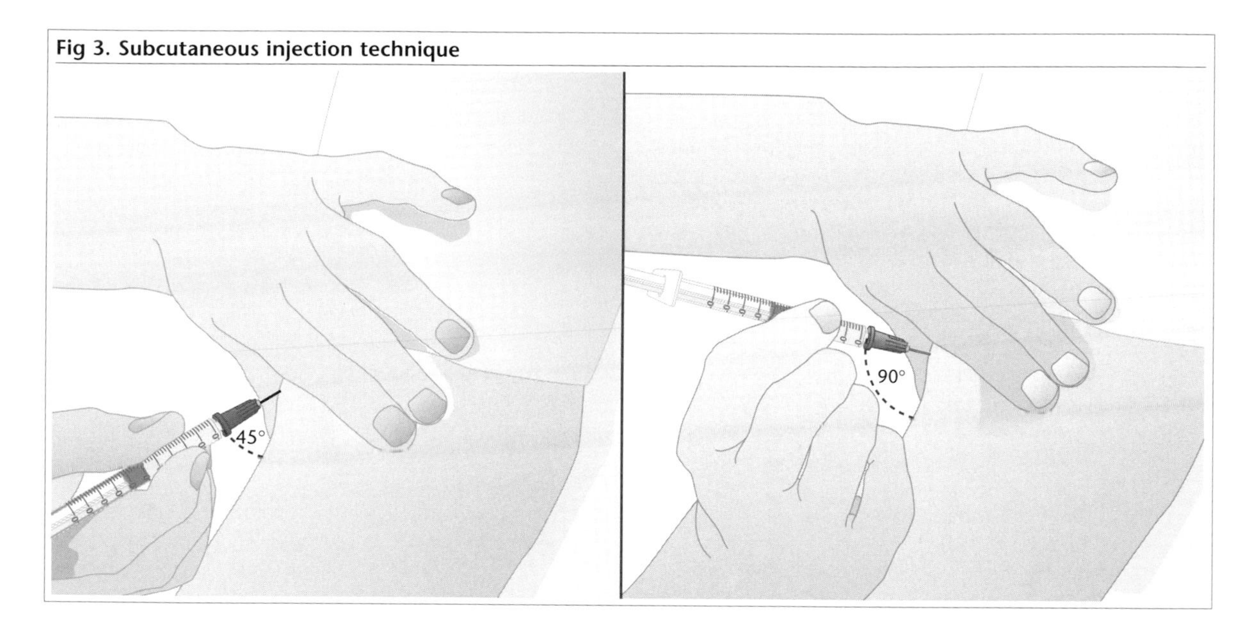

tice in this area, and have access to appropriate sources of expert advice and information.

STANDARDS

When administration of medicines takes place in an institutional setting, for example, a hospital or nursing home, it is imperative that detailed and comprehensive procedures and standards exist in order to encourage safe, legal and effective practice.

Such procedures should take account not only of relevant legal and professional frameworks (for example, the Medicines Act, the UKCC Standards for the Administration of Medicines [UKCC, 1992]), but also of local needs and priorities.

Moreover, such standards should be applicable in all areas of clinical practice irrespective of the practitioners who operate there.

Furthermore, senior practitioners should encourage regular multiprofessional review of such standards in order to identify potential shortcomings. Such review could focus on medicines labelling, legibility of drug administration records, or preparation of intravenous injections and so on.

As the principles of clinical risk management have developed within the health care setting over the last few years, so has the need for all practitioners involved in the use of medicines to work collectively in minimising the risks that are associated with drug treatment.

Such collaboration may range from the development of appropriate documentation to the provision of education and training in medicines related issues. The pace of development and marketing of new drugs and formulations make the task of keeping up to date particularly unenviable.

For practitioners directly involved in drug administration, this poses particular dangers when medicines with which they are unfamiliar are prescribed. The need for caution and diligence is clear.

COMPLIANCE

The administration of medicines in the hospital setting is often made easier in the sense that a high degree of certainty exists on the part of nurses that medicines are being taken or given to the intended patient.

In the community, however, such certainties do not exist, and one of the major drawbacks of our reliance on pharmacotherapy is that either intentionally or unintentionally a high proportion of patients do not take or use their medicines in the way that is intended.

The concept of 'compliance' is notoriously difficult to measure. Estimated rates of non-compliance vary, however, between 30% and 70% of patients treated (Royal College of Physicians, 1984), with older patients being particularly vulnerable.

Compliance can broadly be considered as either unintentional (where the patient may simply forget to take a prescribed medicine) or intentional (where the patient consciously decides not to).

In the latter case in particular, the causes of non-compliance are complex. However, such factors as multiple drug therapy (polypharmacy) , complicated dose regimens (for example, several different medicines, all with differing dose intervals), and unpleasant side-effects are all known to be significant contributory factors.

Patients who are known to be at risk of non-compliance should have their medicines reviewed in order to minimise the influence of the above.

For example, any unnecessary medicines should be

stopped. Those medicines that are required should be given in the smallest appropriate dose and in a form that reduces the number of daily doses to one or two.

Recent research on medicines compliance has demonstrated the importance of the relationship between the patient and the health care provider in determining the level of compliance with prescribed treatment (Royal Pharmaceutical Society, 1997).

Older 'paternalistic' models that have been used to describe the interaction between the prescriber, the patient and their medicines are now increasingly seen as unrepresentative.

In light of this, the concept of 'concordance' has been put forward to describe such interaction as more of a shared process leading to the agreement of the overall aims of any drug treatment and how they are to be achieved.

Throughout this process the patient is able to participate, and is ultimately able to influence the outcome. Achieving concordance between prescriber and patient is thought more likely to lead to higher rates of compliance.

For the patient, a significant part of such agreement depends on the information they have available to inform their decisions.

As notions of consumerism have come increasingly to influence the provision of health care (reflected by such initiatives as the *Patients' Charter* and the emergence of hospital league tables) so patient expectations about the information they require about their medicines has risen.

This has now led to statutory frameworks being established across the European Union under directive 92/27/EEC that require the provision of a standard patient information leaflet with every medicine that is supplied to a patient at any time.

These describe in detail what the medicine is for, its dose and dose interval, its interactions with food and other medicines and possible side-effects.

While the widespread availability of such information is to be welcomed, it is also problematic. Not only are the leaflets densely typed and frequently difficult to read but also the information contained in them may raise concerns that could reduce compliance rather than increase it.

Anecdotal reports in the literature cite the listing of potential side-effects in patient information leaflets associated with corticosteroids, anti-epileptics and acne treatments as having had a direct influence on patients' decisions not to comply with prescribed treatment (Warren and Vincent, 1997).

Such events are, of course, an argument for ensuring that when such information is passed to a patient they have an opportunity to discuss it with an appropriately qualified practitioner who can offer a realistic assessment of a treatments, risks and benefits in terms with which the patient feels comfortable.

It is unfortunately the case that in most situations where patients receive medicines, whether on the ward at discharge, via an outpatient attendance or the GP, the opportunity and facility to deliver such counselling is all too rarely achievable.

The development of medicine self-administration schemes within the hospital setting has become an increasingly popular way of attempting to offset such shortcomings by encouraging patients to manage their own medicines during a hospital stay.

This concept will be discussed in greater detail in part three.

DRUG ERRORS

Just as consumerism has come to influence the manner in which health care services are delivered and measured, so has consumer protection affected the development of risk avoidance and risk management strategies within health care organisations.

The management of clinical risk has particular relevance for practitioners involved in the preparation and administration of medicines, more so in light of the relevance of consumer protection legislation to the use of medicines, and the increasingly litigious environment in which all health care practitioners operate.

Yet the issue of how to deal with medicine-related error within the NHS has all too often been linked solely to disciplinary processes and the attachment of blame.

Such an approach inevitably leads to an under-reporting of error and the potential for harmful practice to go unchecked.

Given the importance of medicines to the overall health care process, the subject of medicine-related error is both poorly researched and poorly understood. Moreover, any analysis of such error has been particularly prone to a uniprofessional approach, which has done little to cast light on the causes of error and, more important, to prevent their recurrence.

A prerequisite for the safe and effective management of medicines in any health care organisation is an open and blame-free approach to the reporting and systematic analysis of drug-related error.

Furthermore, such an approach must be founded on the principle of multiprofessional practice and the adoption of standards that reflect the activity that is being undertaken and not the practitioner who is undertaking them.

Only by the fostering of such an organisational culture will individual practitioners feel sufficiently confident to report their errors and discuss and how they could be avoided.

THINKING POINTS

- **How easy are your local drug administration policies? How useful are they?**
- **What approaches do you employ to help patients/clients take their medication?**

Professional issues

While the development of medicines over the past 30 years has brought vast changes to the way in which ill health is treated and prevented, the main legislative frameworks that regulate the use of medicines throughout the UK remain largely unchanged since becoming statute in the late 1960s and early 1970s.

While the increasing age of these acts is not problematic as such, the development of new and different roles for practitioners with no previous involvement in the use of medicines is presenting an increasing number of legal challenges.

The law now consistently fails to reflect developments in modern day clinical practice.

THE LEGISLATION

The two pieces of legislation of greatest relevance to practitioners involved in the use of medicines are the Medicines Act (1968) and the Misuse of Drugs Act (1971).

The Medicines Act controls the manufacture and distribution of medicines including such details as who can lawfully supply and be in possession of medicines, and how medicines should be packaged and labelled.

It was published largely as a result of the thalidomide tragedy of 1961 and led directly to the establishment of the licensing system that regulates the entry of new medicines into the UK marketplace.

The Misuse of Drugs Act replaced the Dangerous Drugs Act ('DDAs') and controls the import, export, production, supply, and possession of drugs of abuse.

Most practitioners are familiar with its classification of drugs of abuse into schedules of Controlled Drugs (CDs), and the regulations that define how a prescription for them must be written.

Increasingly, this legislation may be replaced or augmented by Regulations and Directives from the European Union.

For example, manufacturers may now apply for European-wide licenses for their products rather than seeking marketing authorisation in each country, and the publication of EU Directive 92/27/EEC places a responsibility on member states to provide patients with patient information leaflets with their dispensed medicines. This directive became law from January 1999.

As yet the UK the government has still to decide how best to implement the directive. However, while much of the law which regulates the prescribing, supply, and administration of medicines is unlikely to be influenced by the EU, there is increasing reluctance on the part of governments to undertake the huge task of revising the Medicines Act.

For practitioners working at the bedside, therefore, there is an increasing sense of frustration that developments in their practice cannot be legally sanctioned.

Fig 4. Example of a patient self-medication sheet

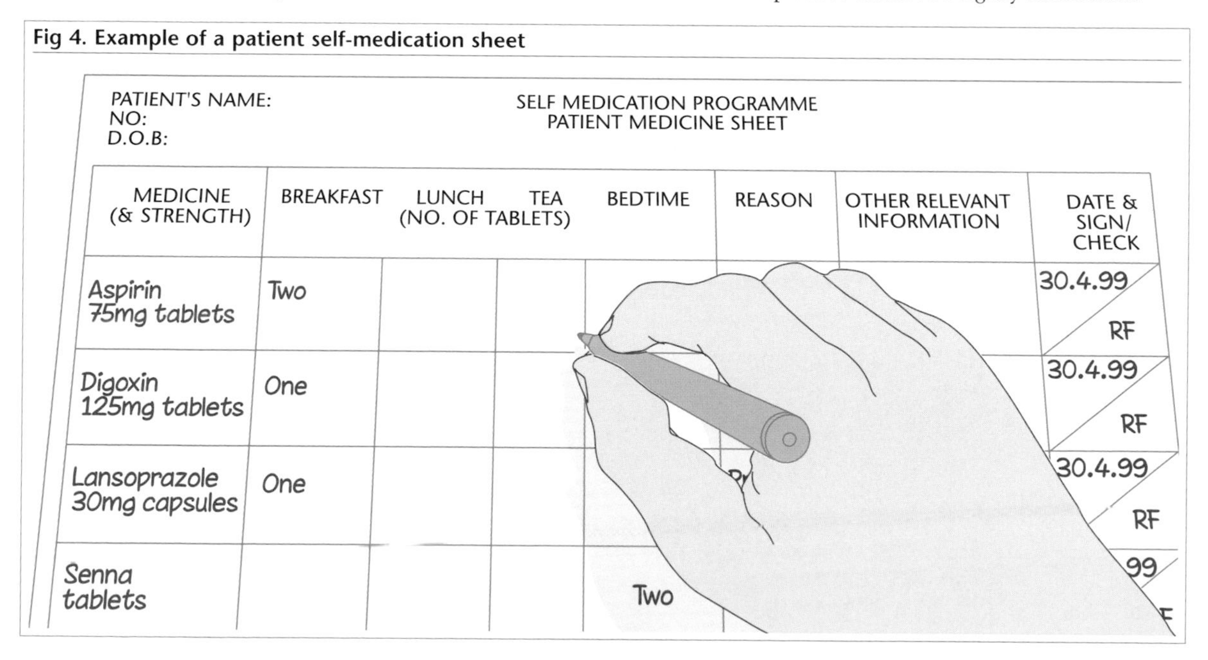

PATIENT'S NAME:
NO:
D.O.B:

SELF MEDICATION PROGRAMME
PATIENT MEDICINE SHEET

MEDICINE (& STRENGTH)	BREAKFAST	LUNCH (NO. OF TABLETS)	TEA	BEDTIME	REASON	OTHER RELEVANT INFORMATION	DATE & SIGN/ CHECK
Aspirin 75mg tablets	Two						30.4.99 RF
Digoxin 125mg tablets	One						30.4.99 RF
Lansoprazole 30mg capsules	One						30.4.99 RF
Senna tablets				Two			99

This may either deter the development of innovative practice or place practitioners at risk of working illegally.

The most compelling example of this relates to the supply and/or administration of medicines under standing orders, or group protocols.

For many years arrangements to allow non-medical practitioners to supply and or administer defined medicines without the written authorisation of a doctor were commonplace in hospitals and GP practices alike, as a means of addressing logistical problems in the prescribing process.

Strictly speaking such arrangements are contrary to the Medicines Act and therefore illegal.

Such frustrations and legal constraints are similarly felt by practitioners seeking to undertake prescribing practice. The March 1999 recommendations of the Crown Committee offer hope of a way forward, however, and in 1998 the committee produced detailed guidance on the creation and operation of group protocols.

The publication of the Nurse Prescribing Act is further recognition of the need for new legislation that can govern and guide practitioners working in new areas.

Self-administration

While the prospects of establishing prescribing authorisation for nurses in the hospital setting remain somewhat uncertain, the key development in secondary care of recent years has been that of patient self-administration.

For many years the standard method of medicines administration in the institutionalised setting has been based on nurses interpreting a prescription and giving the relevant medicine in the required dose via the required route.

The patient's role in such a process being largely passive. The establishment of self-administration as an alternative means of giving medicines is based on the patient being encouraged to play a central and active part in their drug treatment, just as they will be expected to do at home (Fig 4).

The safety and success of self-administration schemes is based on an ongoing nursing assessment that measures the patient's ability to interpret and participate in their prescribed regimen.

Such assessment must initially evaluate whether or not the patient administers any prescribed treatment at home, whether or not they are able to read medicine labels, and whether they can understand dose instructions and so on.

The assessment must also reflect events during the hospital stay.

For example, a patient judged to be capable of self-administering medicines before surgery is unlikely to be able to do so in the immediate postoperative period. Such changes in patient status must be reflected in the patient's care plan, and any indication that the ability to self administer is compromised triggers a return to a nurse administered treatment.

While not a new concept, a number of factors have stimulated hospital practitioners to look afresh at the benefits of self-administration for patients and carers alike.

There is now widespread acknowledgement that traditional methods of medicines administration in hospitals do little to encourage patient compliance and often leave patients at discharge bewildered by a bag of medicines which they may never have seen before, and which they have little idea how to take (Sutherland et al, 1995).

Such methods often lead to significant waste as patients' own medicines are frequently discarded or lost.

By encouraging those patients who are able to administer their own medicines, as they would at home, raises the possibility of identifying education needs and improving compliance.

Moreover, for those patients deemed unable to self-administer, consideration can be given to the problems this may present before discharge.

In many ways the successful cooperation of an extensive self-administration scheme throughout an acute hospital offers insights into the complexities and contradictions of modern medicines management which may, hitherto, have been hidden by the 'drug trolley' approach.

Success requires an acknowledgement that the traditional manner of working does not meet the needs of the majority of patients.

It requires ward-based practitioners to be committed to adopting an innovative approach to their practice. And, arguably most important, it requires a truly integrated multiprofessional approach based on optimising the benefits that patients can gain from the use of their medicines.

Much of the challenge in developing new ways of working and translating them into clinical practice comes from ensuring that the practitioners responsible for delivering them are suitably trained, educated, and competent to meet required standards.

This is particularly true in respect of the supply and administration of medicines. Not only is the rate of change in the pharmaceuticals market place extremely fast (an average of six new products are launched every month in the UK) but also the evidence base that supports the use of medicines in clinical practice is so large and dynamic that maintaining more than a superficial knowledge of it may be beyond the majority of practitioners.

Professional development

Irrespective of their area of practice, all practitioners have a clear professional responsibility to undertake ongoing professional development, but establishing the link between such work and their practical competence in the workplace is particularly difficult.

For practitioners involved in the supply and administration of medicines such competence may relate to the preparation of IV infusions, the assessment of patients for self-administration, the provision of medicines information at discharge or the supply of medicines under a standing order.

Irrespective of the task, it is essential that clear procedures and standards are in place that define the task and how it should be performed.

Furthermore, a system of education, training and assessment must exist in parallel to ensure that practice reflects the standard required and that such standards can be maintained.

The success of such a framework of professional practice development which will depend markedly on the involvement of all practitioners involved in the use of medicines and the extent to which medicines and the extent to which individuals feel able to take ownership of the standards required of them.

NURSE PRESCRIBING

If any one area of health-related law reflects the disparity between statute and clinical practice it is the Medicines Act and the definition of who may lawfully authorise the supply of (or 'prescribe) medicines.

While in the main the Medicines Act places such authority in the hands of medical practitioners, the development of clinical practice within both the primary and secondary care setting has, over the past decade, demonstrated that there is a need for prescribing authorisation to be extended beyond doctors.

This may in part reflect logistical difficulties in the workplace or may relate to the development by a body of practitioners of extended roles accompanied by specialised clinical expertise.

Such considerations may also apply equally to a range of health care professionals including nurses, pharmacists, physiotherapists and dietitians.

Yet while the publication of the Nurse Prescribing Act finally acknowledged the need for such change by granting prescribing authority to a relatively small number of practitioners, (district nurses, health visitors and practice nurses), its lengthy gestation reflected the complexity of issues that surround who should, or should not be able to prescribe and why.

The authority to prescribe brings with it, for example, a requirement not only for diagnostic skills but also knowledge of clinical therapeutics.

Practitioners with no previous prescribing experience may not hitherto have required such skills or knowledge. Extensive training and assessment of competency is therefore a major concern.

Furthermore, other sensitivities surround the task of prescribing such as its implications for the professional status of nursing, its affect on the medical profession, its costs and, ultimately, its affects on patient care.

Such concerns, both legal, clinical, political and economic, mean that extensive nurse prescribing is unlikely to develop at a rapid pace.

THINKING POINTS

- **What are the advantages and disadvantages of patient self-admintsration of drugs in institutional settings?**
- **How far should nurses get involved with the prescription of products traditionally prescribed by doctors? What are the advantages and disadvantages of such an extension of nursing practice?**

REFERENCES

Mallet J., Bailey C.(1996) *The Royal Marsden NHS Trust Manual of Clinical Nursing Procedures*. London: Blackwell Science.
Royal College of Physicians (1984) Medication for the Elderly. *Journal of the Royal College of Physicians;* 18: 1, 7–17.
Royal Pharmaceutical Society of Great Britain (1997) *From Compliance to Concordance*. London: Royal Pharmaceutical Society of Great Britain.
Sutherland, K. et al (1995) Self-administration of drugs : an introduction. *Nursing Times;* 91: 7, 29–30.
UKCC (1992) *Standards for the Administration of Medicines*. London: UKCC.
Warren A., Vincent, R. (1997) Unhelpful information. *Pharmaceutical Journal;* 260: 120.

FURTHER READING

Grahame-Smith, D. G., Aronson, J. K. (1995) *Oxford Textbook of Clinical Pharmacology and Drug Therapy*. Oxford: Oxford University Press.
Mallet, J., Bailey, C. (1996) The Royal Marsden NHS Trust *Manual of Clinical Nursing Procedures*. London: Blackwell Science.
Neal, M. J. (1997) *Medical Pharmacology at a glance*. Oxford: Blackwell Science.
UKCC (1992) *Standards for the Administration of Medicines*. London: UKCC.

Medication

Assessment

When you have read the unit and completed any further reading, you can use the questions below to test your understanding of the topic. Answers can be found on the next page.

1. The study of how the body effects a drug over time is called:

- [ ] 1 Pharmaceutics
- [ ] 2 Pharmakokinetics
- [ ] 3 Pharmacology
- [ ] 4 Pharmacy

2. A drug is said to be an antagonist when it:

- [ ] 1 Mimics the body's natural stimuli
- [ ] 2 Prevents infection from occurring
- [ ] 3 Causes an adverse drug reaction
- [ ] 4 Blocks a normal physiological responser

3. Drug doses are often lower in older patients because:

- [ ] 1 They can't take many tablets
- [ ] 2 Their renal and hepatic function may be reduced
- [ ] 3 Their memory tends to be poor
- [ ] 4 they are more at risk of confusion

4. The extent to which a drug is absorbed via the gastrointestinal tract influences:

- [ ] 1 Whether it can be formulated as a tablet or capsule
- [ ] 2 The side-effects it causes
- [ ] 3 How often it can be given
- [ ] 4 The extent to which it is prescribed

5. A drug for asthma inhaled directly into the lungs is:

- [ ] 1 More likely to be effective than one given orally
- [ ] 2 More likely to cause systemic side effects than if given by mouth
- [ ] 3 More likely to be affected by psychosocial factors than if given by mouth
- [ ] 4 Less effective in older people than drugs given by mouth

6. Adverse drug reactions are thought to:

- [ ] 1 More likely to occur in men
- [ ] 2 Only occur with new drugs
- [ ] 3 Only be of theoretical risk
- [ ] 4 Occur in up to 20% of hospital patients

7. Drugs given by intravenous injection are said to be:

- [ ] 1 Extensively metabolised
- [ ] 2 Poorly distributed
- [ ] 3 100% bioavailable
- [ ] 4 60% bioavailable

8. Which of the following routes of administration carries a risk of systemic side-effects:

- [ ] 1 Topical
- [ ] 2 Oral
- [ ] 3 Rectal
- [ ] 4 All of the above

9. A modified release preparation:

- [ ] 1 Should not be crushed or chewed
- [ ] 2 Is only ever given once a day
- [ ] 3 Has no effect on patient compliance
- [ ] 4 Is less likely to cause side-effects

10. Patient compliance may be affected by:

- [ ] 1 The number of drugs being taken
- [ ] 2 The number of doses prescribed
- [ ] 3 The number of side effects listed in the information leaflet
- [ ] 4 All of the above

11. Nurse prescribing in NHS hospitals is:

- [ ] 1 Legal
- [ ] 2 Illegal
- [ ] 3 Legal if part of a standing order
- [ ] 4 Legal if part of a group protocol

12 **The main legislation controlling the supply of controlled drugs in the NHS is:**

- 1 The Medicines Act
- 2 The Dangerous Drugs Act
- 3 The Misuse of Drugs Act
- 4 The Poisons Act

13 **Self-administration of medicines in hospital is:**

- 1 Expensive
- 2 A good way of reducing nursing costs
- 3 Useful for identifying patients who need help taking their medicines
- 4 None of the above

14 **Standards for the preparation and administration of medicines in hospitals should be:**

- 1 Written by nurses for nurses
- 2 Written by pharmacists
- 3 A local interpretation of legal and professional guidance
- 4 None of the above

15 **The decision to treat a patient with a medicine should be based on:**

- 1 Cost
- 2 The balance of risks and benefits that the medicine offers
- 3 Whether or not they can take tablets
- 4 The patient's age.

ANSWERS

Medication

1: **The study of how the body effects a drug over time is called:**
2) Pharmakokinetics

2: **A drug is said to be an antagonist when it:**
4) Blocks a normal physiological response

3: **Drug doses are often lower in older patients because:**
2) Their renal and hepatic function may be reduced

4: **The extent to which a drug is absorbed via the gastrointestinal tract influences:**
1) Whether it can be formulated as a tablet or capsule

5: **A drug for asthma inhaled directly into the lungs is:**
1) More likely to be effective than one given orally

6: **Adverse drug reactions are thought to:**
4) Occur in up to 20% of hospital patients

7: **Drugs given by intravenous injection are said to be:**
3) 100% bioavailable

8: **Which of the following routes of administration carries a risk of systemic side-effects:**
4) All of the above

9: **A modified release preparation:**
1) Should not be crushed or chewed

10: **Patient compliance may be affected by:**
4) All of the above

11: **Nurse prescribing in NHS hospitals is:**
2) Illegal

12: **The main legislation controlling the supply of controlled drugs in the NHS is:**
3) The Misuse of Drugs Act

13: **Self-administration of medicines in hospital is:**
3) Useful for identifying patients who need help taking their medicines

14: **Standards for the preparation and administration of medicines in hospitals should be:**
3) A local interpretation of legal and professional guidance

15: **The decision to treat a patient with a medicine should be based on:**
2) The balance of risks and benefits that the medicine offers